THINK
AND BE ENLIGHTENED

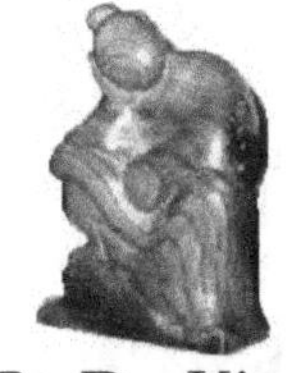

By Dr. King

Dr.King
http://doctor-king-online.blogspot.com

ISBN-13: 978-1974384303
ISBN-10: 1974384306

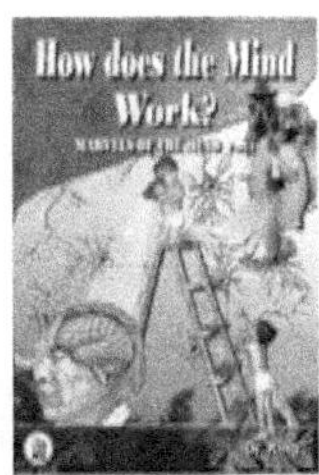

How does the Mind Work?

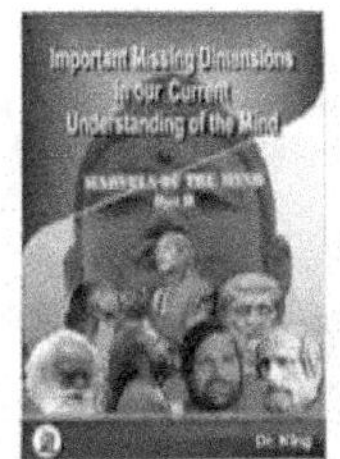

Important Missing Dimensions in Our Current Understanding of the Mind
Dr. King

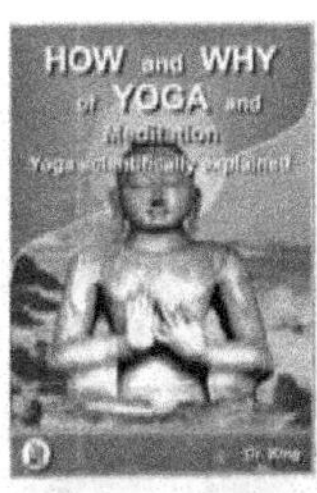

HOW and WHY of YOGA and Meditation
Yoga scientifically explained
Dr. King

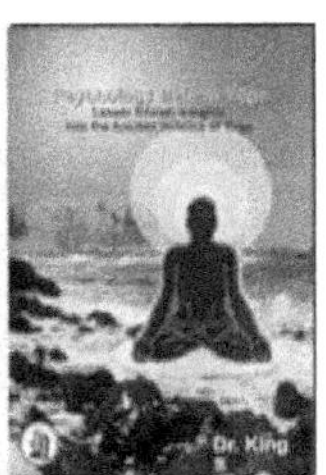

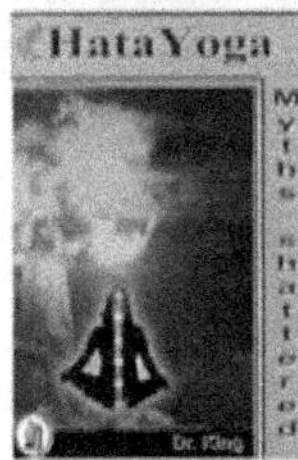

Hata Yoga
Myths shattered
Dr. King

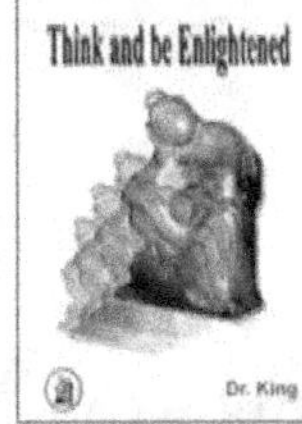

Think and be Enlightened
Dr. King

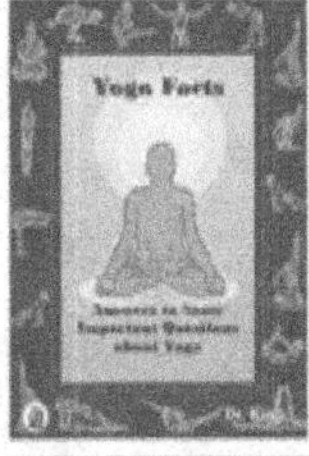

Yoga Facts
Dr. King

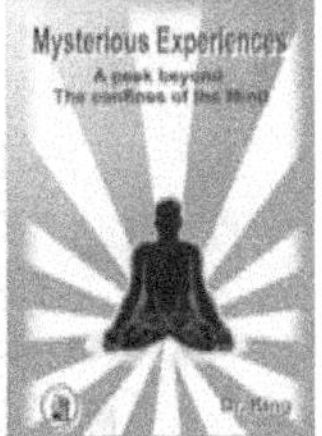

Mysterious Experiences
A peek beyond
The confines of the Mind
Dr. King

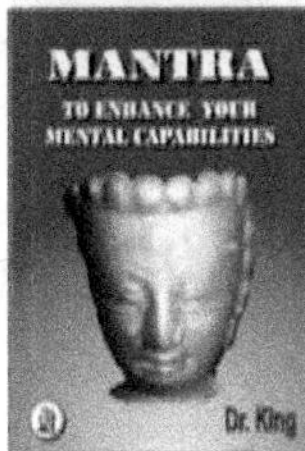

MANTRA
TO ENHANCE YOUR MENTAL CAPABILITIES
Dr. King

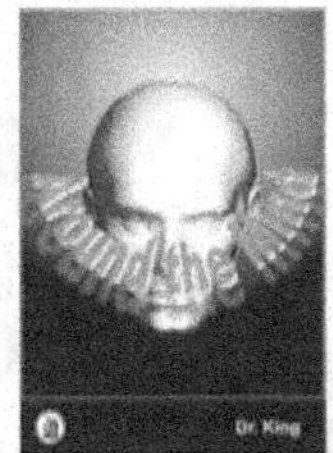

Dr. King

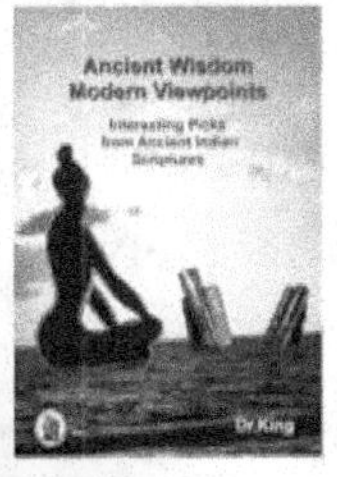

Ancient Wisdom Modern Viewpoints
Interesting Picks from Ancient Indian Scriptures
Dr King

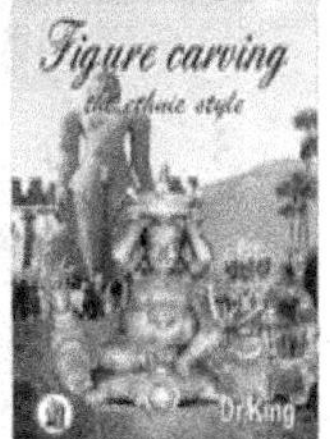

Figure carving
the ethnic style
Dr King

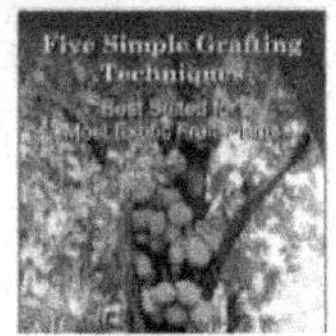

Five Simple Grafting Techniques

Some videos by Dr. King

These videos are free to view. They are also available in 'Free videos' page of Dr.King's blog (http://doctor-king-online.blogspot.com)

1. Yoga scientifically explained
   (https://www.youtube.com/watch?v=k6z un8Ih1nA)
2. Wonderful world of figure carving that you probably never knew about
   (https://www.youtube.com/watch?v=lS2J Vuz9Av0)
3. Mind magic !!!
   (https://www.youtube.com/watch?v=J_K pY12AHUc)
4. Can Yoga be scientifically studied?
   (https://www.youtube.com/watch?v=RR wcZ4Y-yQQ)
5. Brain science behind Yoga
   (https://www.youtube.com/watch?v=ahT 6zlQw6dY)

Table of contents

<u>Inspirational thoughts 67</u>

Prologue

What you see on the cover page is probably familiar to you. It is my logo that I use in all my books, videos, blogs and facebook. I use it to emphasize the importance of thinking.

This book is a compilation of thought provoking posts that I posted on my blog doctor-king-online.blogspot.com over a period of time. Many people found these thoughts very useful. So I thought of putting all of them in the form of a book. Though, these were originally posted interspersed with other posts, here I have grouped and ordered them under different categories to make the reading smooth.

I hope this book will stimulate some thoughts in the reader. Your suggestions and comments are always welcome. Please post them in my blog. You are also welcome to ask any related questions. Use the 'ask me' section (on the right column)

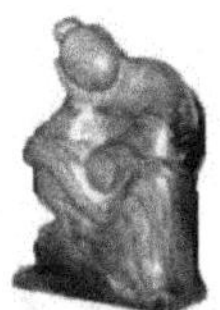

Thoughts on Yoga

1. Yoga timeline (over 3000 years)

One keeps hearing/reading different things being called Yoga. Most people have various notions about Yoga that are quite confusing. So I thought of giving a brief timeline of Yoga (set of practices that apparently resemble the system propounded by Patanjali - a generally accepted source) spanning over 3000 years.

Upanishads – more than 3000 years ago – focus is mainly on meditation including meditation on OM. The purpose is to attain ultimate realization.

Bhagavadgeetha - oldest form believed to have been composed prior to 600 B.C. - in the present form it has 18 chapters each calling itself as Yoga (including Arjuna's remorse). One chapter specifically on Yoga proper, namely "Dhyäna Yoga" very briefly discusses all components of Patanjali Yoga (albeit no Yoga postures as known today). The purpose is ultimate realization and peace.

Tripitaka – recorded sometime during 300 B.C. - these are Yoga like practices taught by Buddha. They have all components of Patanjali Yoga (no Yoga postures known today). The purpose is to free oneself from 'endless cycle of deaths and rebirths (Nirvana)' by proper modulation of the mental processes.

Yoga Sutra of Patanjali – composed sometime during 200 B.C. This is the Yoga proper with 8 components. This composition seems to combine Buddhist techniques in the context of Upanishadic ideas. No body postures as known today. The purpose is to calm down the mind in such a way that one attains ultimate realization.

The following are more recent compositions that laid the foundation for modern Yoga. These are mainly <u>body oriented practices</u> unlike the practices listed above, which are predominantly <u>mind oriented</u>.

Dattätreya Yoga Sastra – composed during 13th century A.D. Emphasizes mainly on various physical techniques meant to preserve 'Bindu' (defined variably as something dripping from head, seminal fluid and so on) and move it up through the spinal column. The word *Hatayoga* (Yoga of force) originated here. Not much on Yoga postures as known today.

Goraksha Shataka – composed during 14th century A.D. by some Yogi belonging to Näth tradition of Gorakshanath. Emphasis and techniques are more or less same as the previous except that the *Kundalini* (a mystic force lying dormant in the perineum) awakening is projected as an end result.

Siva Samhita – composed during 14-15th century A.D. Further builds on previous Hatayoga texts and is an important forerunner of modern Yoga.

Hatapradeepika – composed during 15th century A.D. <u>This is the real basis of modern Yoga</u>. The emphasis is on body and its manipulation to stimulate and raise the *Kundalini* which is the ultimate goal. A short set of Yoga postures is also described, which forms the starting point of modern Yoga.

Gheranda Samhita – composed during 18th century A.D. Builds further on Hatapradeepika and adds more body postures and breathing techniques.

Yoga Upanishads - Believed to be 18th century A.D. and later compositions. Summarize and build on previous Hatayoga texts.

Modern Yoga - Almost all of them are based on Hatayoga described in Hatapradeepika and later texts. Some teachers emphasize on Yoga postures, some on breathing techniques, and some on Kundalini. Improvement of health is the main aim. As compared to Patanjali Yoga, which is <u>mind oriented</u>, this Yoga is <u>body oriented</u> practice. Also, the techniques, operative mechanisms, and goals are all different.

2. Which is the best Yoga?

Nowadays, people have wide options even for Yoga – something like a menu card in a restaurant! Of course, each item comes tagged with a price ;-) How does one decide?

The simple truth is – when you are really hungry, it hardly matters whether you eat in a roadside cheap fast food joint, or while sitting in a luxurious star rated hotel. The purpose is to satisfy your hunger. Well, don't hygiene, health issues and so on matter? For one thing, a cheap place is not always unhygienic, nor a posh expensive hotel guarantees health. So it depends on case to case.

When it comes to Yoga, whether you practice Yoga by putting yourselves in a delicate posture, or whether you breathe in a specific way, or whether you chant a specific mantra, or whether you meditate with exotic mental imageries, it hardly matters. All these ultimately amount to improving your capability to focus and eventually minimize stress.

If you can afford, pay through your nose, and learn how to breathe or how to chant a mantra or do abracadabra! None of these outlets give you any guarantee on safety or its effectiveness or even a decent logical explanation of how it works. So, it all depends on what you can afford and what suits you. Keep your eyes wide open and use your discretion.

One thing is definitely essential – you need to be hungry or else any food is as good or bad as any other ;-)

3. Yogic Law of Exponentials

Many people have asked me – "How long does it take to experience the effectiveness of Yoga?" The simple answer is "it depends!"

For most people effectiveness means stress reduction which is one of the prominent effects of Yoga if practiced properly. Less stress means better health, better performance, peace of mind, and so on. Now, how long does it take?

You probably are aware of what an exponential decay curve is. It is a curve like the one shown in figure.

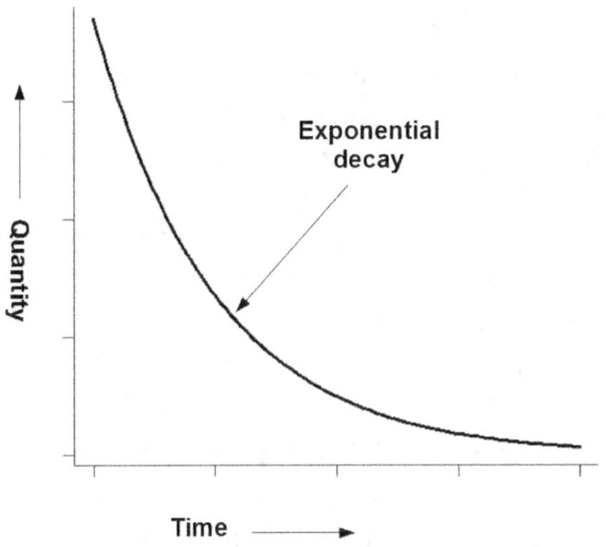

The curve indicates how something decreases over a period of time. The *Yogic law of exponential* is that – "stress decreases exponentially with time, with sustained practice of Yoga". Something like that shown in figure

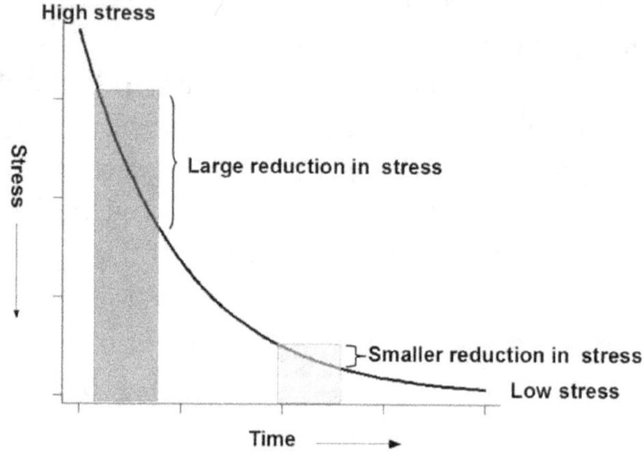

If you start Yoga when you are in a high state of stress, you see quick results as compared to when you start in a relatively lesser stressful state. Not because Yoga is not useful when you are under lesser stress, but simply because the change is perceptible when you are suffering from heavy stress as shown in the above figure. So it depends on how bad your current state is.

4. Yogic hair splitting

Some of my readers have pointed out my 'wrong' usage of the word 'steps' while referring to Patanjali's Ashtänga Yoga as 'Patanjali's 8 step Yoga process'.

Yes. The word *Ashtänga* literally means 8 limbs and not 8 steps. But if you have carefully observed these 8 – there is an order among them, there is succession, there is progression, gradual uplift, and above all, there is an ultimate destination.

> *(1) Yama* and *(2) Niyama* are meant to minimize mental stress and help in calming down the mind;
> *(3) Asana* is supposed to give a steady posture for later practices;
> *(4) Pränäyäma* is supposed to develop mental focus, sitting in a steady/comfortable Asana;
> A focused mind is supposed to result in a state of withdrawal – *(5)Pratyähära*;
> *(6) Dhärana* is to prepare for meditation with a focused mind;
> *(7) Dhyäna* is prolonged dhärana leading to *(8) Samädhi* – a stage where the mind is completely calm.

These are the eight 'limbs' of Yoga. Don't you see order, succession, progression, gradual uplift and an ultimate destination? What are 'steps' in a ladder? They are just that.

Even if you consider Hatayoga, *Asana* is supposed to strengthen the spine (in addition to improving health); *Pränäyäma* is supposed clear impurities in the spinal pathway; *Bandha's, Mu-*

dra's and the like are meant to stimulate the *Kundalini*, which in turn is the precursor to raising the Kundalini through the spinal pathway previously cleared. Raised Kundalini is the ultimate goal. Don't you see them as steps?

So, in addition to seeing literal meaning with a narrow vision, one has to see beyond, taking the complete context in view.

Well, I have seen many renowned 'Yoga' Gurus trying to justify their approach to Yoga taken in a piecemeal fashion – focus only on Asana, or only on Pränäyäma, or only on meditation. They often stress that Ashtänga is not 8 steps but 8 limbs and each limb can be taken up independent of the other as if they are disjoint! I hope Patanjali is listening ;-)

5. Tail wagging the dog!

One of my readers recently complained to me that I give too much emphasis on 'Yama' and 'Niyama' of Yoga. The reader felt that 'Yama' and 'Niyama' are not at all necessary! And laying emphasis on them discourages people from practicing Yoga!

Well, he is not the only one who makes such statements. I have heard great 'Yoga' Gurus also say that.

For people who may not be familiar, let me explain. 'Yama' and 'Niyama' are the first two steps of Yoga that are hardly mentioned by many Yoga Gurus. Simply put

'Yama' means – be honest, avoid hurting anyone, don't desire what does not belong to you, don't amass more wealth than what is essential, and keep your desires under restraint.

'Niyama' means – observe mental and physical cleanliness, be content with what you have, withstand vagaries in life, read things that uplift you spiritually, and have faith in God.

I don't know why someone should be against these basic ethics which in my view are so essential for a healthy society, with or without Yoga, irrespective of your religious affinities! What is making them unacceptable, if any? This reader adds that when someone practices Yoga, automatically he/she becomes honest, ceases to hurt anyone and so on, which essentially what 'Yama' and 'Niyama' are all about.

There is some truth in what he says. But that happens only in advanced stages of Yoga when one attains the ultimate realization. Not in the beginning. So one has to at least attempt to observe these norms if not strictly adhere to them. After all, what is wrong in being honest, kind, content and so on?

I guess it is just an excuse for not doing Yoga in its right spirit.

6. Perplexing 'Yoga' breathing claims

I have read/heard many 'Yoga' Gurus making claims on how 'Yoga' breathing works. I am not sure whether their claims are medically sound.

Many Yoga teachers claim that when you breathe faster and faster, more oxygen gets absorbed by the body and that induces more 'Pranic energy' into the body, giving you health and other mysterious benefits.

But it is well known that the hemoglobin in the blood saturates beyond a level and it cannot absorb more oxygen no matter how fast you try to pump it in. It can only absorb more oxygen when the absorbed oxygen gets depleted at the cells in the body and the blood returns back to the lungs. Considering the natural ratio of roughly 20 breathings to 80 heart beats (fixed by the nature) per minute, it seems that there is always enough oxygen in the air drawn in, to match the absorbing capacity of the hemoglobin. And pumping in more may not help.

But what can happen by faster breathing is the following. Faster breathing may deplete the carbon dioxide from the cells at a higher rate. If you think that that is what gives the benefits, a doctor would probably tell you that depleting carbon dioxide faster can be harmful. It can take you to a stage called hyperventilation, which could adversely interfere with the brain function. Some minimum level of carbon dioxide is essential for the brain to function normally. If the level falls below that level, a person may feel dizzy or it can even be fatal.

My doctor friend suspects that the 'high' often reported during some 'Yoga' breathing sessions may be due to hyperventilation which can make the brain dizzy.

I am not trying to imply that Yoga breathing is not useful. But you don't need to forcibly alter the breathing pace. Just breathe consciously (<u>that is the key</u>) and in a relaxed manner. That would relax your mind as well as develop better mental focus if done regularly, and for say, 20 minutes per day. And it is all free and safe!

7. More is not always better

Some modern 'Yoga' teachers advise their students to perform Yoga postures at a faster pace and do it for a longer duration – more is always better! In fact one of the research papers on Yoga benefits even compares Yoga with some African tribal dance that is supposed to be very strenuous!

I am afraid this is a wrong approach to Yoga. Yoga by definition is a process to calm down the mind. Faster physical activity with associated faster breathing can only agitate the mind and not calm it down. Calming down is necessary for reaping in the health benefits of Yoga. Most research studies indicate that one of the main reasons why Yoga helps is that it has a soothing effect on stress markers.

Instead of trying to do, say 100 Sun salutations (or any other posture), in a given duration, it is always beneficial to do much less number for the same duration and focus more on slow breathing and graceful body maneuvers. That has a higher likelihood of calming down the mind.

But if you are obese or habitually lazy, 'more' may help in burning calories or in keeping you alert. But probably, it is also a fact that overuse of body beyond a limit, can result in wear and tear and cause health problems. So, next time when your Yoga Guru tells you that 'more is better', ask him/her to explain why. That is the only way.

8. Views of "Who am I Swami" (Ramana Maharshi)

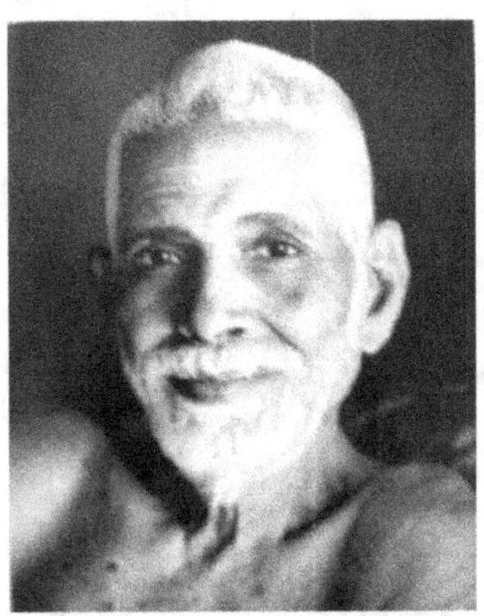

One of the greatest Yogis in recent times was Ramana Maharshi (1879-1950) who lived in Tiruvannamalai in the South India. He had definite views on Yoga and other realted philosophical aspects.

i. Who am I? Swami – on Hata Yoga

You probably have read about this spiritual man from southern India, made well known in the west by Paul Brunton through his book "Search in secret India". His actual name was Ramana Maharshi (1879-1950). He acquired the name "who am I? swami" since he used to advise people who came to him to enquire who they really are. According to him this was the most direct route to ultimate realization or rather removal of ignorance.

Recently someone sent me a book (actually a compilation of conversation with the swami) which the sender said has lot in common with some of the statements I have made in some of my books on Yoga. Actually, I had never read about Ramana before, except the one by Brunton. So I was curious. This book with more than 700 pages had many statements by Ramana about Yoga. These statements were markedly contradictory to what is popularly known about Yoga today and the statements made by several well known modern Yoga teachers. Here is one snippet.

"They (the hata yogis) think that after purifying the 72,000 nadis in the body, sushumna is entered and the mind passes up to the sahasrara and there is nectar trickling.

These are all mental concepts. The man is already overwhelmed by world concepts. Other concepts are now added in the shape of this Yoga. The object of all these is to rid the man of concepts and to make him inhere as the pure Self - i.e., absolute consciousness, bereft of thoughts! Why not go straight to it? Why add

ii. Who am I? Swami – on Pränäyäma

Pränäyäma or Yogic breathing is considered to be one of the important aspects of Yoga practice. Modern Yoga teachers give mysterious explanations about how it works. For example, in one of the interviews the renowned Yoga teacher B.K.S Iyangar says something like this.

> *"Pränäyäma is not just breathing in and out. It is directing the subtle and invisible energy called Prana (life force) through the nostrils in such a way that it hits against a specific nerve centre"*

Most modern Yoga teachers give similar explanations about this important Yoga technique. But none explain it logically nor give exact references supporting their statements. And you don't find these in Yoga Sutra of Patanjali either.

Here is what Ramana has to say about Pränäyäma.

> *"If life is imperiled the whole in-
terest centers round the one point, the saving of life. If the breath is held the mind cannot afford to (and does not)*

29

> *jump at its pets - external objects. Thus there is rest for the mind so long as the breath is held. All attention being turned on breath or its regulation, other interests are lost... ......The mind improves by practice and becomes finer just as the razor's edge is sharpened by stropping."*

Interestingly, I gave a very similar explanation about Pränäyäma in my book "How and Why of Yoga and Meditation". I was a bit nervous at that time since my views differ from popular beliefs and there was always a chance of someone getting offended. I was not trying to show that popular beliefs are wrong. My intention was to separate logically explainable parts from the apparently mysterious practices so that we can make progress. And now, after reading Ramana, I feel lot at ease!(thanks to the reader who sent me the book on Ramana)

iii. "Who am I? Swami" – on paths to salvation

(Continued from previous post)

As the name with which he is well known suggests, Ramana's emphasis had always been the path of enquiry, namely "who am I?" But in general he suggests four paths.

1.   Path of enquiry
2.   Path of devotion
3.   Path of Yoga
4.   Path of Hatayoga

In all these paths Ramana says that the underlying principle is the same – stopping the mind and its activities. But Ramana hastens to add that stoppage of the mind does not mean complete stoppage. The awareness has to continue even after stoppage of other mental activities. Otherwise, he points out, a person in deep sleep, a person who is in coma, or a person who is unconscious in general, would all have attained salvation! In none of these cases the awareness persists though the mental activities have stopped.

This is yet another point I have discussed in my book "How and why of Yoga and Meditation", where I have equated "awareness" to the activity of the "attention system" in the brain. This system should not be shutdown but should be in a highly active (while most of the cortical activities have stopped) state to attain self realization.

Let me briefly discuss the four paths suggested by Ramana.

1.Path of enquiry

This is Ramana's pet path. Ramana says that when someone constantly indulges in the enquiry – "Who am I?" all other thoughts in his mind gradually stop and he will reach a stage of samādhi. This is when the ultimate self realization is attained and according to Ramana, that is the direct path to salvation.

2.Path of devotion

In this path, Ramana says that one focuses his mind on an external object such as God, Guru and so on, and expresses devotion to that object. Though Ramana disapproves the existence of separate God or Guru (Ramana believes in just the soul and nothing else), he says that in the initial stages such devotion helps one to stop mental activities since the mind is repeatedly focused on God or Guru. But gradually this focus turns inward and finally leads to self realization where he realizes that "He" himself is both the God and Guru.

This is yet another point where there is amazing similarity between Ramana's views and what I have discussed about devotional singing in my book "How and why of Yoga and Meditation".

3. Path of Yoga

By Yoga, Ramana means the Yoga system laid down by Patanjali and not what we know today as Yoga. Ramana fully agrees with Patanjali's definition of Yoga as "Yoga is about restraining the activities of the mind". And the process naturally leads to samädhi and ultimate self realization.

4. Path of Hatayoga

Today, most people take the words Yoga and Hatayoga as if they are synonymous. But not Ramana. All through his conversations Ramana directly or indirectly makes light comments about Hatayoga, though he repeatedly says that he does not wish to criticize any path. The first post in this series namely "Who am I? Swami – on Hatayoga" says it all.

Another strange recent development is - equating Yoga postures or asanas to Yoga, though originally Patanjali talks about none of the asanas propagated by modern Yoga teachers. On several occasions when people ask Ramana about his opinion about asana, Ramana intentionally or unintentionally evades direct answer. Sometimes he uses the word asana to mean meditative postures such as the lotus posture and says that they are useful during meditation or while doing Pränäyäma. Sometimes he uses the word asana to mean just the seat (in Sanskrit language that is what it means) on which a person sits during meditation, and says that whether it has to be on a deer skin, layer of kusha grass etc. (these are the seats some Yoga teachers recommend), is immaterial. He talks lightly about strange explanation given by these teachers for the use of a particular type of seat.

Ramana's final word about Hatayoga is that - those who cannot follow the first 3 paths probably get benefited by Hatayoga, though he repeatedly says that it is a roundabout path which has to ultimately lead to the first three paths!

Though I have tried to show that there is not much of support for asanas (as they are known today) in ancient texts, I have discussed some proven health benefits of these asanas in my book. I have also discussed the possible reasons for the same.

iv. "Who am I? Swami" – on ultimate reality

Knowing the ultimate reality has always been the quest of all intellectuals from time immemorial. Each philosopher has his/her own version of this reality. What does Ramana have to say about this ultimate reality?

Ramana's often repeated assertion is that in the ultimate sense this world does not exist! What we perceive as world around us is "just a creation of the mind" and as such it actually does not exist!

Ramana gives the example of deep sleep when we are totally unaware of any world around us though we know that we exist. The world "appears" only when we wake up from our sleep and our mind once again starts functioning. Similarly, in samādhi - deep state of meditation (when the mind has stopped functioning), once again the world disappears. The obvious conclusion of Ramana is that world exists only when the mind functions. Or in other words, it is the creation of the mind.

People who are familiar with ancient Indian philosophy at once recognize similarity of this view with that of Vijñānavādi Buddhists, or the philosophy of Gaudapāda – grand Guru of well known Advaita proponent Šankara.

In my book "Some important missing dimensions in our current understanding of the mind", I have discussed in detail how Gaudapāda puts forth his argument and even claims support from Upanishads. In that book, I have also discussed how Šankara later disagrees with this theory, and ridicules the Vijñānavādis in his commentary on Brahma sutra – one of most important ancient texts on Veda.

One of the readers of my book strongly objected to my view that Šankara disagrees with this theory even though I had quoted profusely from Šankara's commentary. This reader felt that it is "a commonly accepted fact that Šankara propagated the same philosophy put forth by Gaudapāda".

It is interesting that one of the visitors to Ramana points out this fact (that Šankara has refuted this view in his commentary), Ramana refuses to change his view and continues to say that world is only a creation of the mind and it does not exist!

I wonder whether the words in the Brahma sutra commentary attributed to Šankara were introduced later by his followers to escape from the allegation that this view is borrowed from the Buddhists. Since Ramana quotes heavily from Yoga Vasista – a supposedly 10th century composition (which was believed to have been continuously modified till 18th century), is it likely that Yoga vasista was composed based on Šankara's original views which were modified later on by his followers ? – I am only trying to hazard a guess.

On my part, I find it difficult to accept Ramana's/Gaudapäda's views on this since I feel

- ▶ Upanishads don't support this view as Gaudapäda tries to show.
- ▶ Šankara's views expressed in the Brahma sutra commentary are genuine unless proven otherwise.
- ▶ It is possible to logically show that the deep sleep analogy given by Ramana, or the dream analogy given by Gaudapäda are not foolproof.
- ▶ It does not make any sense to have any discussion or enquiry if the entire thing is only nonexistent.

I have discussed all these issues in my book mentioned above. As always, my intention is not to show that all these great men were wrong, but to question till satisfactory answers are got.

9. Do you meditate?

You probably are thinking of meditation as something that you learn by attending some classes, or by reading some books; where you sit cross legged, with your eyes closed, trying hard to calm down your mind.

No. Meditation is not just that. You can turn anything you do throughout the day into meditation. In fact, you can be meditating all the time!

When I water my plants I carefully watch around the plant to see if the soil is too dry or is it too wet. I water accordingly. I feel the plants gracefully swaying as if to say "thank you". I talk to them and gently pat on their back.

When I dig a hole in the ground for a new plant, I enjoy the feel of the fresh moist soil as I dig it out. I take in the aroma. I observe the tiny creatures hiding beneath, and gently lift and set them aside so that I don't harm them.

Whenever I get some time, I engage myself in carving. I carve wood since wood carving demands the most concentration. A small lack of focus can result in a mistake that is hard to correct. My carving subjects are normally monk figures. My friend tells me that the figures I carve, though not perfect, have a serene look on their face. Since you are carving monks, your mind gets filled with serene thoughts and that serenity in turn gets reflected in the pieces you make.

I was reading Tipitakas (ancient Buddhist texts). One of them describes the last days of Buddha. Buddha went through severe illness as the end approached. But even at that stage, it is said, Buddha was calmly observing each stage of the approaching death, the feelings they created, the last moments of his life. And that is meditation!

10. As many Yogas, so many theories

Nowadays we come across whole lot of things propagated as 'Yoga'. Almost all of them trace the origin to Patanjali. Interestingly, there are equally many theories about what these 'techniques' can achieve and how they work. I was curious and thought of recording them. Here are some.

Theory 1.

Yoga basically involves modulating the mental activities so that the mind calms down completely by a step by step process. A completely calm mind enables one to realize the ultimate.

This is the theory propounded by Patanjali (300 B.C.) in his Yoga sutra. Even ancient Buddhists had a very similar explanation to their meditative techniques that also work like Yoga. Incidentally, I have also tried to explain Yoga on similar lines in the light of modern neuroscience in my book "How and Why of Yoga and Meditation – Yoga scientifically explained".

Theory 2.

Yoga involves channeling the cosmic power called 'Kundalini' from 'moolaadhara' (in the pelvic region) to 'sahasraara' in the brain, passing through various 'power centers' (called 'chakras') that lie along the spinal cord. This is achieved using various Yoga techniques. When this power reaches its destination, the person who practices Yoga gets ultimate realization.

This is the theory propounded by Hatayoga Pradeepika (15th century). Many modern Yoga teachers who propagate variants of this 'Hatayoga' talk about very similar theories. Some of them even attribute its origin to Lord Shri Krishna in Bhagavad Geetha (apparently even before 300 B.C.) . But as far as I am aware, the theory in Bhagavad Geetha is closer to the one propounded by Patanjali.

Theory 3.

The Yogic breathing acts like bellows that kindle the fire in the lower abdomen. As a result the impure and thick blood in the heart starts boiling. When this blood boils, impurities in it get separated in the same way as impurities separate from molten gold. These impurities are expelled though sweat that is produced during Yogic postures. Since the root cause of ill health is these impurities, Yoga makes the person healthy.

This is a theory supposedly based on some little known 'ancient' text. This theory forms the basis of many modern Yoga variants that seem to be quite popular. These systems give utmost importance to Yoga postures and breathing.

Theory 4.

Our body is encircled by currents of cosmic forces. When one moves the hands and other limbs in the process of performing various Yoga postures, these currents get directed to flow into the body. Their entry into the body charges it up and makes it healthy.

I am not sure what the basis of this theory is, but I have read some Yoga proponents give this theory. May be influenced by some Chinese concepts.

Interesting!!

11. Whither Yoga?

It is once again – Yoga day. Many of my Indian friends feel proud of the fact that the entire world has acknowledged India's one of the greatest contributions to the world namely Yoga.

But when I see how this word Yoga has been torn to pieces and made into a totally ill defined system, from what originally was a very well defined science, I feel sad.

Just the other day, I was talking to my Indian doctor friend. He is a highly qualified allopath, but nevertheless open to any system of medicine. I asked him why he does not try Yoga for his long time diabetic condition. One of the most popular Yoga teachers in India today, namely Baba Ramdev claims that he has recorded evidence of curing hundreds of thousands of diabetic patients just by making them do Kapalabhati – one of the 'Yogic breathing techniques' he has been trying to popularize. I asked my doctor friend's reaction to these claims.

My friend simply smiled and said "in that case, Baba Ramdev should be awarded a Nobel!"

Very true. If curing diabetes were that simple, world would have been too grateful to him and got rid of one of the most menacing health problems these days.

Baba Ramdev very confidently asserts that any disease can be cured or even prevented by simple breathing techniques he is propagating in the name of Yoga. The irony is that none of these techniques were ever talked about by the well known ancient proponent of Yoga namely Patanjali. But Baba Ramdev projects them as if they are part of Patanjali's Yoga system!

Probably, there is a silver lining in the cloud. People like Baba Ramdev would help in drawing wider attention to Yoga from more and more people. More attention means more critical analysis sooner than later. Ultimately that would separate chaff from grain. Hope so.

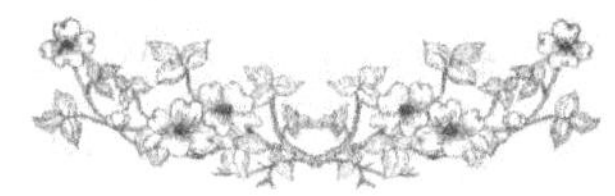

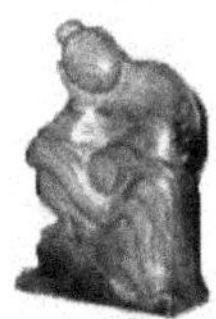

Thoughts on Indian philosophy

1. Yoga of action

Many a times we fail in our well intended efforts to do something and we get put off. Sometimes the setback discourages us so much that we hesitate to make any more efforts. In this context, following well known words of Krishna in Bhagavad Gaeta may be kept in mind.

"Your jurisdiction is restricted to making best efforts. The results are not always under your control. So, never get put off by the failures and cease from making further efforts.

None can totally abstain from action even if she/he wishes to. The inherent natural instincts force one to keep doing something. So indulge in necessary actions, while keeping yourself detached from success or failure.

Even if you have reached a stage where you don't need to do anything, you still have to keep doing right things at least for the sake of setting an example for other people who may otherwise resort to inaction or wrong action. If that happens, you will be guilty of misleading them.

(Selected verses from chapters 2 and 3 of Bhagavad Geetha adapted suitably)

2. Yoga of devotion (Bhakti Yoga)

When I read the holy Quran for the first time, what drew my attention the most was the concept of total unquestioning surrender. Surrender to God or some supreme power is something you can find in almost every religion. Even the supposedly atheist Buddhism stipulates surrender to Buddha as a prerequisite to accepting Buddhism ("Buddham saranam gachchami").

In Bhagavad Geetha, Krishna says

"Always think about me. Always be my devotee. Always surrender to me. If you do that, I will take care of your welfare and safety.

I don't expect anything from you other than total surrender. Whatever you offer to me – be it a flower or a fruit or even a leaf or mere drop of water – I accept it as long as it is offered with purity of mind and total surrender.

So, whatever you do, whatever you eat, whatever you practice, offer all that to me (i.e. do them for my pleasure). Even if you abandon all other paths, I will protect you from all miseries. Do not be afraid"

Here, Krishna can be replaced by any other God or Supreme Being.

PS: For those of you who probably find it difficult to accept the concept of God, I would like to draw your attention to the fact that many a times the results of faith do not necessarily depend on the existence or otherwise of the object of faith. Besides, Krishna never said - "Don't do anything but just depend on me". He said - "Keep doing what you need to, but offer that to me and take solace that I will take care of you".

(Selected verses from chapter 9 and 18 of Bhagavad Geetha adapted suitably)

3. The "Ða","Ða","Ða" story

Once the Gods, Demons and humans went to the Brahma (the ancient Indian concept of supreme power), seeking advice.

To Gods, the Brahma said - "Ða".

The Gods took it as "Ðama", meaning - "control your excessive sensual desires",since Gods were by nature extemely sensual.

To Demons, the Brahma said - "Ða".

The Demons took it as "Ðaya", meaning - "be merciful towards those who are weaker than you", since Demons were cruel by nature.

To humans, the Brahma said - "Ða".

The Humans took it as "Ðäna" - meaning "be generous towards those who are in need", since Humans were greedy by nature.

Those were the good old days. Today, we seem to have a little bit of Gods and Demons in us in addition to being humans. So we need to do "Ða, Ða, Ða"

* Story from ancient Upanishads

Note: "Ða" is pronounced as "thu" in t he word "thus".

4. Tat Tvam Asi

This is a series of posts based on the well known discussion in Chändogya Upanishad (part of Säma Veda, believed to have been recorded more than 3000 years ago) regarding ultimate truths.

i. Do you know 'that'?

What is it 'that' I am talking about? It is 'that' after knowing which you know everything; it is 'that' after hearing which you have heard all; it is that after understanding which there is nothing more to understand.

Does any such thing exist?

That was exactly the question young Swetaketu asked his father.

Swetaketu had spent 12 years in his residential school, away from home, and had learnt whatever was there to learn. But no teacher ever taught him 'that' which apparently makes all other knowledge superfluous.

Swetaketu was arrogant. He thought he knew everything. And this arrogance is what his father wanted to eliminate by pointing to him that knowing the essence is more important than knowing the details. If you know the essence, you know everything; or else you know nothing. How is that?

We will see that in the next post.

ii. Understand the fundamentals

There are probably infinitely many things in this world. Each is different in its own way. Each has a different use. Each has a different property. But all these infinitely many things are made of 3 fundamental particles – electrons, protons and neutrons. These 3 particles in different combinations and different configurations form all that that exists in this world.

You can spend your entire lifetime to understand each of the things in this world. Or if you understand these three fundamental particles and their properties, you almost know everything in this world. Rest are just the details!

Ancient Indians also talked about three fundamental things that formed everything in this material world. These three things are *sathwa, rajas and tamas. Sathwa* has no mass but it only has potential energy. It is like the proton. *Rajas* also has no mass but it has kinetic energy. It is like an electron. And finally, the *tamas* is all mass and nothing else. It is like the neutron.

The ancient Indians believed that once you know these three fundamental elements that form the entire material world, you know everything.

Well, almost. What is it that we left out?

We will see that in the next post.

iii. Matter is not everything

Science says that everything is material. There is nothing else. In that case, why is a living person living and a corpse a dead body? A living body as well as a dead body are both made up of the same set of basic elements. But one is alive and the other is dead. Why?

Ancient Indians (so also Greeks as well as other ancient civilizations) said that it is the soul that makes the difference. A soul makes an otherwise dead body a living body. A body minus the soul is dead!

So this world is made up of three fundamental elements in various combinations and configurations, plus the soul. It is not just the elements alone.

But how did this world come into existence? That is what our current science is not clear about.

We will see that in the next post.

iv. Something can't come from nothing

No matter what science says, ancient Indians were clear that something cannot come from nothing. What was that 'thing' which this world came from?

For want of a better word, ancient Indians called that thing as *Sath* – which literally means existence. This world came from *Sath* and not from nothing. So 'in the beginning' there <u>was</u> this *Sath* that created or took the form of 'everything' that we see around – the world, the beings in it, and so on.

How does one infer that?

We will see that in the next post.

v. Trace the cause from the effect

If you want to know the origin of the universe, keep tracing back the cause, starting from the effect. You will eventually reach the starting point.

For example, you see a huge tree with hundreds of branches, thousands of leaves and so on. How did this tree come into existence?

The leaves sprouted from the branches; the braches from the trunk; the trunk from the root; the roots from the seed. The seed may be very tiny but it is what brought up the massive tree. You can't see the tree in the seed, but you can infer it by back tracing.

Now, how did the seed sprout into a tree? It got the energy from the soil, water and sunlight. And from where did soil, water and sunlight come from?

In this way, you can back trace each and everything in this world and infer the ultimate cause. The ancient Indians inferred the penultimate cause to be three basic elements – sathwa, rajas and tamas - and the soul. And the ultimate cause that gave rise to these is the 'existence' itself, which they called *Sath*.

There is another way to infer this.

We will see that in the next post.

vi. Forward trace instead of back tracing

In the previous post we back traced to infer the fundamental cause for this universe. There is one more way that can lead you to the same conclusion.

Instead of back tracing, trace forward.

Supposing you have a dying man. Observe him carefully. Gradually, his ability to see, hear, feel and so on cease. And finally he dies. His body is still there but he is dead. Why? Because the soul has left the body.

Now observe the dead body. If you leave it as it is, it decomposes and finally gets transformed into the same basic elements from which it came. Essentially, you are left with basic elements and the soul from which the entire forward process started. And we have seen in earlier posts that it is the *Sath* that is the root of these elements and the soul.

What it means is that *Sath* is the prime cause of all existence as well as the ultimate destiny of all that came from it. The world emerges from *Sath* and finally gets back to *Sath*. Or in other words, there is an endless cycle of 'creation' and 're-absorption' of the worlds. What we have been talking about as the 'the beginning' is just one point in this endless cycle. And the 'creation','re-absorption' are only changes in name and form.

But all these explanations don't convince. We never see this happening - the same basic cause operating behind the diversity we see all around. How are we sure? The boy Swetaketu also has the same doubt. His father gives further illustrations.

We will see that in the next post.

vii. More ways to sink in the fundamental truth

In the previous posts we saw the origin and final destiny of the universe that we see around. But Swetaketu was still not convinced in spite of his father reasoning it out the way we did in previous posts. So, father gives more analogies to sink in the truth.

He asks the son to bring a seed of a huge Banyan tree. The tree is huge, diverse but it is a fact that such a huge and diverse tree sprang out from a tiny seed. But, if one breaks open the seed, one can never see the tree inside, however much one magnifies it. But the tree did emerge from a tiny seed. So it is possible for a vast, diverse world to emerge from a subtle cause like *Sath*.

How is it that we don't see this prime cause operating? The next illustration that the father gives is as follows. The father asks Swetaketu to dissolve some salt into water. Once dissolved, the salt is not visible, but its existence can be inferred by tasting the water taken from any part of the solution. So also, the *Sath* pervades all that that emerged from it, but still remains imperceptible to casual observation.

But how is it that all these things finally return back to the *Sath* at the end of the 'creation-re absorption' cycle? Swetaketu's father gives the simile of the rivers that finally merge with the sea and become one with it. Before merger, each river was different, had its own name and form. But post merger, they all lose their separate name and form and become one with the sea. They came from the sea, and finally merged into the sea.

So what is 'that' truth we started with in the beginning?

We will see that in the next post.

viii. 'that' which one needs to know

We started this series of posts with a question whether there is anything after knowing which we know everything; after hearing which we have heard everything. Or in other words, what is the essence of all the diversity we see around us as the world and our individual existences?

The Upanishad (Chändogya Upanishad chapter 6, sections 1 to 16, "The *story of Swetaketu*") says that this essence is as follows.

Whatever subtle thing from
which this entire world came forth

*has also made things in this world
alive by entering them in the form of
individual souls. And in essence,
'each one of us is nothing but that'.
This is the ultimate truth.*

Anyone who has 'realized' this fundamental truth has understood everything and there is nothing more to understand. All our worldly knowledge is only an elaboration of whatever that ensued from 'that'. And so, once we know 'that' we know everything.

This is the well known *Advaitic* (non-dualistic) statement *'Tat Tvam asi'* – 'That thou art' - 'You are That'.

PS: Incidentally, the same statement has been interpreted differently by the *Dwaitis* (dualists) in consonance with their point of view..

5. Poornamadha....

i. Strange Mantra

There is a strange mantra that is normally recited in the beginning of many Upanishads (philosophic parts of ancient Indian scriptures, namely Veda).

Literally translated, the mantra says

*"That is complete. This (too) is
complete. (This) complete has come*

56

> *from (that) complete. When complete*
> *is removed from complete, what re-*
> *mains is also complete"*

On the face of it, it sounds absurd. If something is complete, how can it remain complete when something is removed from it!

Scholars have given varieties of interpretations to this apparently absurd mantra. Many chant it with religious fervor without bothering much about its meaning and implication. But it does have very profound meaning.

In the subsequent posts, I am going to use this mantra to explain several such seeming absurdities, be it in mathematics or philosophy.

Let me start next with a case in mathematics.

ii. Strange Mathematics

Normally, when we remove 'something' from something else, the original 'something' will become smaller. That is elementary mathematics.

But mathematicians have a concept called 'infinity' – something that has no limit, something that is not finite. Take for example, the total number of whole numbers. There are infinitely many of them – you name any number, there is another number which is larger than it.

What happens when you remove something from infinity? Will it become smaller? No, not always. It depends. Consider for example, the total number of numbers. As we saw earlier, there are infinitely many of them. What happens if we remove all even numbers from this set of numbers? You are left with infinitely many odd numbers.

You started with something that was infinite. Removed something which was also infinite (there are infinitely many even numbers!) and what you are left with was also infinite – infinitely many odd numbers.

That means, infinity minus infinity need not be zero! It can even be infinity. Or if you ponder a bit, it can be zero or finite even!

That is strange mathematics. Isn't it?

Even in the area of philosophy there are such strange apparent paradoxes. Let us see that next.

iii. Strange Philosophies

Two of the highly intriguing Indian Philosophies in recent times (I am talking in a wide time frame) is the Advaita philosophy propagated by Šankara and the Dvaita philosophy of Madhva - both from Southern India, both being staunch supporters of ancient Vedic ideologies.

Strangely, the philosophies advocated by these two great masters were diametrically opposite! – Or at least they appeared to be so, on the face of it.

Very briefly, Šankara's view was that the multiplicity seen in the world is just an illusion.

There are not infinitely many things in this world! In 'reality' there is only a single entity in the world namely, the indefinable Brahma or Ätma.

While his counterpart, namely Madhva, held the view that multiplicity is the reality and there is not one, but three categories of things in this world, and each of them is real. None of these is identical, nor are they even comparable.

The interesting point to note is that both these scholars claim the Upanishads to be the basis of their assertions. Each has his own reasoning and logic to prove his point. Each has written volumes of commentaries to support his views and each has wide following.

How can the same source (Upanishads) give out such seemingly contradictory views? Strange isn't it?

To sort out this seeming contradiction, probably we need to look at the source i.e. the Upanishads themselves. That is what I am going to do next.

iv. Root of the mystery

In one of the well known Upanishads, namely the Chändogya Upanishad, there is a description of how this world came into existence. Let me summarize the relevant verses as follows.

"In the beginning, there was nothing but 'That' alone that existed.

And 'That' wished to be many. It took the form of 'Tejas' (bright light). This 'Tejas' too wished to be many and it took the form of 'Äp' (water). This 'Äp' in turn took the form of 'Anna' (nutriment)"

What is interesting is even after taking these various forms the original 'That' remained as it was. Explaining the 'creation process' further, the Upanishad explains how each of these three forms – bright light, water and nutriment – combined among themselves and resulted in the formation of several entities each distinct in its own way. Then the Upanishad says

"Having taken so many forms, 'That' entered each of them in the form of 'Jiva' (soul) and separated 'name' and 'form'"

So, in this way, the single entity that alone existed in the beginning 'became' many things/beings that we see around us as 'world'.

But how is that possible? How can one entity become many and still remain as it was! We will see this in the next post.

v. Our space-time limited world

We live in a space/time limited world. Here, no entity can exist in more than one place 'simultaneously'. Similarly, no two things can occupy the same space at the same time.

The consequence of this limitation, that we take for granted, is that an entity cannot have more than one form at the same time. Also, the form dictates the capabilities of the entity. For example, water can either be liquid – as water, or solid – as ice, or gaseous – as steam, at different times but not at the same time. And when it is liquid it has different properties and uses as compared to when it is in solid form. So these names and forms make them different, though the contents can be one and the same.

What if we remove this space/time restriction?

In such a situation, a single entity can be liquid, gaseous, or solid at the same time: probably, many more things. Though they appear to be many different things, they all are indeed the same thing.

With this relaxed restriction on existence, let us trace back our discussion to previous posts.

vi. Multiplicity in the universe is real

Recall the Chändogya Upanishad description of the creation of the world that we discussed in an earlier post. Originally there was a single entity. But that single entity took different names and forms and 'became' many.

Once it became many, each form has its own limitations and properties. In that respect no two forms are identical. An apple is not same as orange – each has a different shape, color, looks, taste and so on. So also, any two individuals – you are not identical to me. We are different in our own ways. Are we at least same as that 'original' thing from which we all came from? Definitely not. The original 'That' had neither form, nor any limitations.

This is the Dvaita philosophy of Madhva. He said – "no two inert ('Jada') things are identical, nor are they same as any living being ('Jiva'). Neither are they comparable with 'That' ('Paramätma'). Similarly, no two living beings are identical, nor any of them are comparable with 'That'".

In essence, there are five kinds of differences between three categories of entities namely 'That', soul and inert things. i.e.

1. difference between inert things,
2. difference between inert and living beings,
3. difference between inert things and 'That',
4. difference between living beings ,
5. difference between living beings and 'That'

This is the so called 'Bheda väda' (philosophy of differences) or commonly called Dvaita philosophy of Madhva. Since the original 'That' was real, each of the other two categories of entities is also real. So, not only the world but also the diversity in the world is real.

Does this mean that the other philosophy, namely that of Šankara is wrong? Let us see that in the next post.

vii. Multiplicity in the universe is only apparent

Recall again the Chändogya Upanishad description of the creation of the world that we discussed in an earlier post. Originally there was a single entity. But that single entity (simultaneously) took different names and forms and 'became' many.

No matter what forms and names the original 'That' took, the fact remains that each of those forms are all 'That' in the essence. The names and forms may be different. It is a case of simultaneous coexistence of the same entity in many forms. In our space/time limited world view, such a thing is difficult to comprehend. But let me give a simple example to illustrate this point (this is only for illustration, please don't stretch it beyond limits)

Assume that there are multiple movie theaters adjacent to each other, each running different movie with the same actor playing the lead role. In each movie, the actor plays a different role – in one he may be a drunkard, in another he may be a wicked man, in yet another he may be a saint and so on. The role is dictated by the story line of each movie and the actor plays exactly as per the script – the name and form he has taken.

At the same time the real actor sitting somewhere, may neither be a drunkard, nor wicked, nor a saint. He is in no way bound by the story line of the movies he has enacted. For a viewer, the same actor appears differently. But behind all those diversity of roles, it is the single actor who is playing the roles. The differences are imposed by the story lines of each movie.

So if we ignore the space/time limitation of our perceptible world, it is not too difficult to understand that behind all this seeming diversity, there is a single entity that appears differently.

This is exactly (well, almost), the Advaita philosophy of Šankara – "Brahma (the name used for 'That') alone exists, the diversity is just apparent (Mithya) "

Let us move back a step and see the original strange mantra with which we started and see how all these things mesh well. That will be the next post.

viii. Demystifying the strange mantra

Recall the original strange mantra we started with.

> *"That is complete. This (too) is complete. (This) complete has come from (that) complete. When complete is removed from complete, what remains is also complete"*

If we equate 'that' to the original 'That' which alone existed in the beginning (recall the Chändogya Upanishad creation story) and 'this' to our perceptible world we see around, including us, the meaning of this apparently strange mantra becomes almost clear.

This world came from 'That'. And as per the Upanishad, even after this world came out, 'That' remained as it was. 'That' did not get transformed into 'this'. It took more forms and coexists with all those forms.

There is no doubt about the fact that the original 'That' was limitless or 'complete'. But each of the forms taken by 'That' is definitely not limitless and complete. Each has its own shortcomings.

If that is the case, how does the above mantra say that 'this' is also complete?

We probably have to see each of the entities in 'this' sans the name and form it has taken.

What do we see there? 'this' is same as 'That'. This is what exactly, many Upanishads say – when all names and forms are dropped, 'this' becomes indistinguishable from 'that' or in some way 'this' merges with 'That' in the same way "the rivers merge with the sea when they finally lose their individual names and forms". Before merging, each river had a name and its own characteristics such as speed, breadth, length, force and so on. But once they merge with the sea, there is no river but just the sea.

This is also the momentary experience one gets in advanced stages of meditation or samādhi. When the identity with the body is overcome, the limited 'I' becomes universal 'I" which is limitless.

So, 'this' is also 'complete' in reality.

PS: I am aware of possible objections some staunch Dvaita adherents may have to my explanation. I am only trying to unify diversity in views and see sense in various Upanishadic verses, and great philosophies of these masters whom I hold in high esteem. After all, in the domain of 'infinity' our 'limited' algebra does not work as we saw earlier.

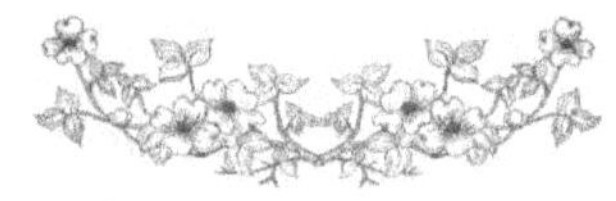

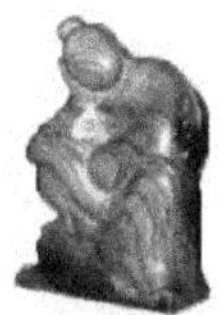

Inspirational thoughts

1. Two views

There are two views

i. First view

- One is that human beings are inherently perfect but imperfection is something that is superimposed on them.

- The other is that human beings are inherently imperfect and need to evolve to perfection.

There are people who categorize the former as "typical eastern view" and the latter as "western view". Or probably as Hindu verses non-Hindu view. But that is not so.

Ancient Greeks considered "psyche" as the driving force behind all living beings. And this Psyche is the most perfect and holy. That being the case, there is no way we can be inherently imperfect. Imperfections, if any, are added onto something that is inherently pure and perfect. Pythagoreans even went to the extent of saying that these imperfections can be "cleansed" by mathematical reasoning.

Even the Bible says that God created human beings "in His likeness". So, God being perfect, there is no way his likeness can be inherently imperfect. As per Bible, it is the Satan who brought in blemishes on what would have been otherwise perfect.

Ancient Indians considered all beings as forms of God who is by nature perfect. In fact, there are several verses in the Upanishads (parts of Vedas) that describe how the one and only 'Ätma' (the Upanishadic equivalent to God) replicated itself to take on several forms (living and nonliving). The imperfections we see, are either illusions (as per Šankara's Advaita), or something that are superimposed on what is inherently perfect. An Upanishadic sage prays

> *"The golden pot is covered by darkness. Oh God! Shine your light so that the darkness is driven away and the pot's full glory is made visible"*

Here the "golden pot" being referred to is the individual who even though perfect, appears to be imperfect due to darkness (superimposed blemishes).

So, there seems to be unanimity among the ancient thoughts – whether eastern or western, Hindu or otherwise – that human beings are inherently perfect and holy. If anything, we need to remove the imperfections that are superimposed.

As against this view, the other view is that we are basically imperfect and we need to 'become' perfect. I will talk about that view in the next post.

ii. Second view

The other view we were talking about was that

"Human beings are inherently imperfect and need to evolve to perfection."

Most of our current thinking revolves around this view.

An evolutionary theorists says that 'we' started as unicellular organisms, evolved into more perfect animals, further, as intelligent apes and finally as human beings who are the most perfect of all. We may continue to evolve into more perfect beings.

An anthropologist would tell us how we evolved from primitive, barbaric and perhaps nomadic tribals into more refined and more capable, cultured races with a well defined societal structure, following rigid norms for peaceful coexistence.

A social scientists may explain how a basically 'animal like' creature namely human beings can be molded into more refined being by setting up appropriate rules and regulations. All of us are criminals by nature, but adopt a more 'civil' way of life for the fear of punishment. Stricter and stricter enforcement of laws is the only way to make us better human beings.

The clergy would term each of us a sinner and would urge us to repent and pray to become better human beings.

All these stem from the assumption that we are inherently imperfect and we need to 'become' perfect by refinement.

Now the question is which one of these two views is right? Are we inherently perfect and have become imperfect or that we are inherently imperfect and need to become perfect?

2. Knowledge belongs to everyone

"Preach that to every one from the roof top, which I whispered into your ears, and the ones I told you in the darkness, announce it to everyone in broad daylight. No, there is no secret to be hidden from anybody"

-- Jesus Christ

3. Faith versus scientific attitude

Faith is an inalienable part of life. Faith asks no questions. It just accepts things. Intellect has no place in faith.

There is really nothing like blind faith – all faiths are blind if you choose to categorize them that way.

Acceptability of any faith depends on its long term consequences and not on its validity.

Any faith is acceptable as long as it does not have adverse repercussions.

One needs to be flexible to alter one's faith when it is found to be harmful.

i. Faith versus scientific attitude (continued 2)

Faith is beautiful. But ...

There is no guarantee that faith always takes us forward.

In contrast, scientific attitude provides some guarantee about moving forward. It is like oaring the boat in a known direction rather than just drifting along with the tides.

Scientific attitude is a systematic approach to life.

When it matters, scientific attitude is preferable to faith.

ii. Faith versus scientific attitude (continued 3)

Faith stems from the emotional aspect of human beings, whereas scientific attitude is driven by intellect.

Emotions are essential for survival, whereas intellect is needed for continued existance and evolution.

It is not sufficient to merely exist. One needs to evolve further. That makes both faith and scientific attitude part of life.

4. Do we need to be more analytical?

Many a times we let our decisions guided by others.

- We buy a product based on some TV or news paper advertisement.
- We buy a book based on the number of reviews the book has got.
- We accept someone as a Guru based on the crowd he pulls.

How often do we sit back and think whether all these people could be manipulating our decisions for their own benefits?

- An ad could be a false propaganda or presentation of partial information.
- The reviews could be 'self sponsored'.
- A crowd pulling Guru could be a smart marketer.

We need to look at the facts rather than opinions. We need to be guided by reasoning rather than emotions.

5. Speaking the truth

- ✓ One should speak the truth.
- ✓ One should speak in a way that does not hurt anyone.
- ✓ One should avoid telling harsh truths.
- ✓ So also untruth even if it pleases someone.
- ✓ This IS the eternal code of conduct.

-- Ancient lawmaker Manu.

6. Who is a real teacher?

Someone who teaches you things or the one who enables you to learn on your own ?
As an old Chinese adage goes

> *"one who teaches you how to catch fish is greater than the one who feeds you with fish"*

So also a teacher. He needs to enhance the comprehending capabilities of the student rather than feed him with readymade knowledge.

7. Truth of truth

I came across a self claimed rationalist blogger vociferously declaring that belief in God is just a superstition since no such God exists. In response, another self claimed Guru counseled that the existence of God cannot be argued upon, but should be just experienced.

Which of these conclusions are correct? Actually, as far as truth is concerned, it is always relative. There is no absolute truth. If you are a person who can see the world, the entire world is colorful. But, for a born blind person, it could be sound full or even touch full but never colorful.

Most of the time, what is true is not that important but in what way it affects us is important. Unfortunately, all truths have an associated weight. If two truths have the same weight, you can accept either of them.

If a Baba says that by breathing in a particular way, blockage in your arteries, even if it is 90%, can be cleared, there may be some truth with non zero weight in his statement. But there is high risk of having heart attack if you accept his truth as against the counsel of a cardiologist who has recommended angioplasty. You may still die of heart attach even after angioplasty but the chances are less. The reason is that the weight of Baba's truth is much less than that of the Cardiologist's truth. So, it is the weight which is important when it matters.

In rest of the cases, you are free to accept any truth depending on your choice.

8. Balance is the key

Life is full of uncertainties, full of problems. One way to get around this situation is to improve the circumstances by minimizing uncertainties and reducing the problems to the extent possible. All our achievements, innovations revolve around this approach. This approach has a global effect and helps humanity as a whole.

However, the main catch in this approach is that no matter how much we toil, the uncertainties don't completely vanish nor our problems. So it is a continuous struggle between nature verses human endeavors. Added to this, more we minimize uncertainties and problems, more we get sensitive to even traces of them. So, our problems continue.

The other approach is to train our minds in such a way that we become indifferent to these problems and we develop equanimity. In such a state, no matter the uncertainties or problems, they don't affect us at all. This is the approach taken by Buddhism.

Even this approach has shortcomings. Firstly, this approach is totally individual centered. It has no global effect. An individual who can train the mind in such a way, can escape the hardships; but what about those who cannot? The majority of humanity would continue to reel down under uncertainty and misery. We remain passive spectators to all suffering and uncertainties, and there is no moving forward.

What is needed is a balance between these two approaches – keep improving the situations in the best interest of all as well as ourselves, while trying to keep the mind calm and unperturbed.

9. An ancient coin mint dated 200 B.C.!

That was a joke we made about my childhood friend who claimed that he has a coin which was actually minted 200 years before Christ! When asked how he was sure of that, my friend replied that the date 200 B.C. is written on the coin!

Every country, religion, always had people who cleverly faked things to imply that they are actually very ancient and tried to take advantage of that. Most of the time, it is almost impossible to prove the genuineness of such an artifact.

Recently, I came across a bunch of 'supposedly ancient Indian scriptures' each claiming to be part of ancient Vedic literature (2000 B.C.). Some of them talked about Yoga which is one of my fields of interest. Many of the ideas discussed in these scriptures seemed to have lot in common with the ideas propagated by many modern Yoga Gurus, though none of these find mention in the generally accepted Yoga bible "The Yoga sutra" by Patanjali. I could see many telltale marks of intentional fabrication, though it is very difficult to pin them down.

While a western scholar would labor hard to fix historical credibility of any purported ancient scripture, most traditional Indians give no importance to historicity and their judgments are guided by faith alone. But such an approach has its own associated long term adverse consequences.

What is the right approach? Yes, historicity is important. But since it is almost impossible to judge in many cases, we probably have to take a via media. There are other factors that can help in accepting or rejecting such documents. (See my earlier post on how we should look at such documents.) After all, old is not always gold!

10. Enjoy but without over indulgence

An ancient Indian philosopher namely Chärväka is supposed to have said

*"one should enjoy at any cost,
even by borrowing from others"*

This seems to be our aim in life these days. Everyone wants to enjoy without bothering about the long term consequences.

Recently I was very much pained to know the death of three young brothers in my neighborhood. All three died one after another in short intervals of time. They were young, well educated and my interaction with them always gave me the impression that they were nice and well behaved. The cause of their untimely death was over drinking. They were hospitalized several times, the doctors had warned them in advance, and they themselves were intelligent enough to know their folly. But they could not give-up drinks.

It is not just drinks; our craze for enjoyment these days makes me wonder where we are headed to?

In this context, I remember another Vedic seer's sane advice (in Ïshävästa Upanishad)

> *"One should aspire to live and enjoy in this life for full 100 years. Protect yourself with detachment (never overindulge). Never covet other's possessions. This is the only way to avoid wrong doing."*

11. Right approach to education

We often see many people around us who cling to false beliefs that give them short term peace of mind, but misery in the long term. The question is – do we need to tell them what is 'right' so that they avoid ensuing misery?

Educating the ignorant is necessary but we need to be cautious to ensure that the advice is taken in the right spirit and it really helps them.

I remember an old story where a group of monkeys gather around a heap of red seeds on a cold winter night, hoping that the red seeds would warm them up, the way glowing embers do. It never happens that way. A small bird sitting on a nearby tree, that was watching the foolishness of the monkeys, tries to advise them on their folly. The monkeys ignore the bird's advice and kill the poor creature for questioning their intelligence. But they too die due to exposure to severe cold conditions since the red seeds don't help them in any way.

If the monkeys had heeded to the bird's advice, they could have saved their lives. The fault of the bird is that it was giving advice to ones who are unprepared to accept it. Secondly, the bird was merely pointing out the mistake without suggesting any alternative.

12. Real Social Service

If the miseries of a fellow being brings tears into your eyes, go ahead and help that person. But remember, a better way is to do something to change the situation that has brought that misery. After all, you just cannot help each and everyone, however much you may wish to.

13. Extraordinary claims need to be supported by extraordinary evidence

Human beings seem to have an innate craving for mysterious things. And many clever manipulators cash on this weakness. We often tend to forget that extraordinary claims need to be supported by extraordinary evidence. Making tall claims without supporting evidence – either logical, or literature based, or experimental – is not only misleading but can even be dangerous. Magic rarely happens and we need to be on the watch to avoid being duped.

14. How to be an achiever?

Rather than getting into philosophical discussion on "Who is an achiever?", let me get down straight into a simple method that almost always works.

1. At the end of the day, just jot down how you spent the whole day, what you did from time t1 to time t2, and so on. Be honest, don't skip anything and don't try to gloss over.

2. Look at the list of things you did. And ask yourself the following questions –
   - "Was that really needed?"
   - "Could it have been done in a better way?"
   - "Does it really benefit me in the long run?"

You don't need to make any changes or build any strategy for improvement. It just happens automatically. Do this for a month or so, sincerely, and to the best of your abilities. And you are sure to see changes. And once you get used to it, you don't even have to do this exercise anymore!

What actually happens is that you become more conscious of what you do. And that is the key. More often than not, we are poor time managers, we do things mechanically or unmindfully and the result is poor achievements. Being conscious of anything you do, by itself is one of the great meditation practices.

15. Isn't life too beautiful?

During my occasional visits to a chain store near my house, I used to meet this nice elderly white lady who used to sit at the checkout counter. Her heavily wrinkled face revealed her age as at least late eighties. I always wondered what forced this lady to work in a store at that age!

One afternoon, while I was checking out my things, we observed a small crowd gathering in front of a high-rise building just outside the store, across the road. A person who just entered the store at that time told us that someone jumped from the top floor of that building and committed suicide.

I could see the old lady's face paling out with the shock. With tears in her eyes, she softly exclaimed – "honey, isn't life too beautiful to end like that? What's happening to this world?"

16. What you experience and what IS, need not be the same!

Nowadays, I see some popular Gurus making their supposedly 'mysterious experiences' as their USP. They urge their prospective disciples to believe what they experience as the ultimate reality.

Though I have discussed some mysterious experiences in my book *"Mysterious experiences –*

<u>*A peek beyond the confines of the Mind*</u>", I have all along held the position that even if it is a fact that you have experienced something unusual, what you think you have experienced need not be true.

A lunatic may experience lot of things. His experiences are real in the sense he has gone through them. But what he has experienced need not be true. A drug addict may feel as if he is flying in the air. But in reality he may be just lying down on his couch!

Somebody's mysterious experiences by themselves do not prove him to be a mystic or a self realized person. It just means that he has experienced something for which he has no explanation. There may not be anything 'spiritual' about it. It could be just some weird happening in the brain ;-)

It is not always necessary to interpret things we don't understand as 'spiritual' or for that matter, as 'realization'.

17. Can you play a string less guitar?

Probably you think it is absurd – playing a guitar without strings?! Not really. Let me tell you a small story.

Once an opponent challenged Buddha whether he can be as happy as the great King Bimbisar, who was wealthy, had all power and comforts, whereas Buddha had nothing except for a begging bowl.

In return, Buddha asked the man whether the said king can remain happily for a week, few days or even a day doing nothing physically, mentally. Buddha declared that he can easily do that. The essence of Buddha's words is that happiness is not really in worldly pleasures or comforts, not even by being engaged in bodily or mental activities. It is something beyond.

If you have ever tried to remain all alone, not interacting with anyone, not reading or writing, nor watching anything, not even thinking, even for a day – you probably would realize how impossible it is. You can't get pleasure without physical/mental involvement – without tweaking the cords of body and mind.

But believe me, it is not just Buddha, but you too can experience immense bliss incomparable to physical/mental pleasures – you too can play string less guitar!

18. Do your duty

If you wish to bring some positive changes in the society, don't be deterred if results don't meet your expectations. Often they don't. The results are not always under your control. But it is better to attempt than remain an idle spectator.

> *"The field of one's operation is*
> *restricted to only performing one's*

19. "Let all positive things come to us from every-where"

So goes one ancient Vedic saying (Rig-Veda 1.89.1). That is the epitome of openness. On the other extreme, we have people who are closed to anything outside their limited boundaries and prefer to live in an imaginary world.

Almost every religion claims that it comes straight from the God's mouth. Each patriot is too proud of his/her ancient tradition and be-lieves that it is flawless. But it is rarely the case.

The right approach is to accept anything good, no matter from where it comes, and ignore inevitable shortcomings. Every religion, every country has something special to offer. And ac-cept it without bias. But make sure that your openness does not lead to stupidity and gullibili-ty.

Moreover, if you are in a position where your word has influence over the masses or if you have taken up a role to bring positive changes in the society at large, you have the **responsibility** to draw attention to negative things as well, and try to explain why they are not acceptable. Your silence can mislead others. But you always need to put your views in such a way that people see the reasoning behind your views and accept them willingly.

20. World is one big family (Vasudhaiva kutumbakam)

> *The petty minded persons differentiate between "my people" and "other people". But a person with noble character always considers the entire world as one big family.*

-- old Sanskrit saying

21. Miracles everywhere! Keep your eyes open.

I vaguely remember the two books that I read long long ago. One by Paramahamsa Yogananda ("Autobiography of a Yogi") and the other by Swami Rama ("Living with Himalayan Masters"). Both these are more of anthologies of miracles than strictly autobiographical.

Though I was a bit skeptical while reading these two books, they did keep me engrossed. I have seen many people – highly educated, as well as lay – very much impressed by the miracles described in these books and needless to say that these books succeeded in further arousing their appetite for miracles.

But we often tend to ignore those miracles that keep happening just in front of our eyes and look for them elsewhere! After all what is a miracle? It is just an unusual happening that baffles us and we fail to fully understand it.

Take for example, the birth of a child. Just a lump of flesh that hangs upside down in the mother's womb for nine long months, gets forced out through a passage too narrow for it to pass through, the passage suddenly expands to accommodate the exit, the extreme pain that the mother experiences during the entire process that she later cherishes as a sweet memory, the tube that nourished the fetus all through gets detached on its own when the baby comes out, the baby takes in a puff of fresh air for the first time in its life, and starts feeding on the fluid that gets spontaneously produced in its mother's breasts....... Each event is unusual, one that baffles us, and all the same we fail to understand how such a thing could happen. Isn't that a miracle?

Miracles keep happening every second, everywhere, wherever we look around. We just need to keep our eyes open. No need to look for them elsewhere.

22. Path is not really important. But ...

Imagine that there is a hill and you would like to have a view of the surrounding from the top of the hill. If you are energetic, you may climb the hill. Or you can take an uphill path that ultimately takes you to the top. You can ride on a mule and make your journey easy. Or if you can afford, you can even take a chopper and reach the top almost without effort.

But did you notice something? No matter how you reached the top, the view from the top is one and the same!

The saints, prophets, monks and rishis of every religion – whether it is Judaism, Christianity, Islam, Buddhism or ancient Indian – all reached the same top, some through faith and devotion, some through meditation and some through intellectual enquiry. All of them had a glimpse of the same view no matter how they reached there. The path they took is just a matter of suitability and convenience.

So don't give too much of emphasis on the path you take. Choose what is suitable to you, the one you can afford, the one you are comfortable with. If you are sincere enough, you will ultimately reach the same top no matter the path.

But watch out. You may come across people on your way, people who have never reached the top, who don't know the path, but who merely pretend to have known, have reached, and take you on a long trip round and round the hill, never ever reaching the top!.

23. One step at a time

Many a time things look altogether formidable. What we try to do looks almost impossible. Right now I am trying to carve a life size figure of a monk. The log I am using weighs almost as heavy as me! It is quite hardwood. I may have to chisel out almost half the wood. All that I have is a simple chisel. Can I do it? I never tried a figure of that size before.

Based on my prior experience on similar occasions, I just concentrate on "now". I tell myself – "I need to chip off 'this' small part of the log". I go on doing it chip at a time without bothering about the complete task on hand. It works!

Simple approach. But it almost always works.

24. Back to basics

Now-a-days we see people who are busy all the time. They have no time for anything. The result is stress and tension.

While someone resorts to some "XYZ Yoga" to relieve stress, someone does a "3 minute cure-all mediation/mantra chant" to relax. We chase the wild goose in all wrong places. Do we ever pause and ask

- What are we busy for?
- What is it that we want to achieve ultimately?
- Is the busy schedule imposed on us or
  was that self created?
- Do we really get what we want, after all
  this grinding?

Think about it!

25. One magic bullet for all ills!

I have often wondered whether there is any single most important thing that can bring a massive change in the way we all live in.

Let us analyze a bit. Do you realize that most
of our decisions in life are driven by what others
do? We rarely take decisions based on self
judgment but depend upon 'mass perceptions'.
While this approach has lot of pluses to its cre-
dit, this probably is the single important cause of
most perils, in my view.

One of my blog posts received highest
views. I was quite perplexed since the post does
not have anything that makes it so popular. On
some analysis I found that for whatever reason,
once this post happened to get maximum clicks
for some time and it reached top of 'popular
posts'. From then on, anyone who visited my

blog was curious to know what this 'popular post' is all about and they clicked it. More people tried that, the post continued to remain on top and the cycle repeats!

I have seen authors who openly admit that they themselves buy their own books periodically, to keep the book on top of the sales ranking. Higher the sales ranking, more people will be tempted to buy it and the cycle continues! Same is the case with 'sponsored reviews'.

On a larger perspective, most governments in many democratic countries come up not because the leaders have proven track record, but purely based on the mass opinion they have managed to establish. Especially in countries where political awareness is low, people vote a party not because they have full information about the leaders in that party but because everyone else does it!

So, what is the magic bullet?

Enable one to judge himself/herself rather than depend on other's opinions.

That will be the single most important contribution one can make to bring in a phenomenal change. Teach them to judge rather than to follow someone else.

26. Don't discourage questions

When we are too small, our elders often restricted us from doing several things without giving any valid reasons. Probably, that was the only way since we were too young to understand reason.

But I see many Gurus, discouraging questions, saying that they are hindrances to spiritual growth. They probably forget that any religion, or practice that puts down a list of do's and don'ts <u>without explaining the reasons</u>, has invariably deteriorated into a self destructive dogma.

It is the duty of a Guru to develop the student to a level where he/she can decide for himself/herself, rather than impose rules that are made to be accepted without questions. Questioning is necessary for a smooth growth.

In this context, I am reminded of the most crucial sentence in Bhagavadgeetha (ancient Indian scripture). After answering all the questions of Arjuna, Krishna says (Bhagavadgeetha 18.63)

> *"I have explained to you the most profound knowledge. Now you ponder over it completely and do as you feel fit (....Yathä ichchasi tathä kuru)"*

27. Mere scholarship is not enough

I often come across highly qualified people falling an easy prey to fake Gurus or mysterious practices. There does not seem to be any relation between their scholastic achievements and their ability to judge things especially when it comes to so called spirituality. On the other extreme, I see self claimed Gurus who are apparently well read, failing to exhibit conviction and deeper insight.

The reason is – when it comes to spirituality, it is not enough to read. One needs to ponder over what is read, grasp the finer aspects of it and finally meditate on what is understood. Not only that, one needs to live a specific way of life. Only then one can get complete insight.

28. There is still hope

I often get disturbed by the rampant violence either in the name of racism, religious faith or just any other intolerance that we see around us these days. I keep wondering whether humanity is moving towards its annihilation!

I have spent varying periods of my life in various countries and interacted with people of different nationality, race and ethnicity. Without fail, I have always found the same humane face everywhere. May be I was lucky. But what makes me hopeful is that majority of humanity is sober. They just believe in "live and let live" policy. It is just that a few odd ones create all the trouble and they get the most attention.

Nature, I firmly believe, has built in mechanisms to preserve itself. So, in spite of occasional failures, it always recovers and moves on.

29. Know your strength

Sometimes we tend to overlook our strengths and brood over our weak points. It is not arrogance to be aware of our strengths, but it is necessary at times.

It was a hot summer afternoon. I wanted to dispose off some vegetable and fruit peels. Normally, I feed some stray cattle that happen to come that way. I went out of the house looking for some prospective needy. Found a big stray bull standing under a tree. It was quite big and scary. I did not dare go anywhere near it. If it so wished, it could toss me around just by a slight movement of its hefty body.

But I did not want to waste the peels either. So, I hesitatingly moved towards the bull.

Surprisingly, the bull started running away from me! It was quite scared of me, though I was no match for its strength!. After a bit of enticing and cajoling. it stopped and looked at me. Only then I could throw the things at it.

The bull was quite strong and I was no match for it. But it did not know that!

30. New Year resolution - A suggestion

When we were kids, most of us used to ask lot of questions. But as we grew, we stopped asking questions and started accepting whatever others said or did. And we stopped growing!

Ask questions and continue to grow. Otherwise, you will just age, year after year.

Best wishes for a growth full New Year!

31. Desires etc. are not bad per se

Most ancient religions considered desires as bad. Especially, the eastern religions consider desire ("käma"), anger ("krödha"), greed ("löbha"), possessiveness ("möha"), conceit ("mada"), jealously ("matsara") as six enemies of mankind.

But just think about it. Are these not essential, in some form or other, for our very existence?

Without sexual desire probably the beings cannot continue to exist in the form of progeny. Without desire for happiness, none of our achievements are possible. Anger is definitely needed to defend ourselves and our companions from an aggressive offender. It is greed that makes us save for tomorrow to take care of future uncertainties. Without possessiveness, we cannot probably take care of our people and belongings. Conceit encourages us to do better in anticipation of recognition. Jealousy also indirectly coaxes us to make progress so that we can be better than others.

So, none of these are our enemies per se. They are all essential and probably inalienable parts of our life. But when do they become hindrances?

Let see that in the next post.

i. Be the master and not the slave

In the previous post we saw how our six instincts namely desire, anger, greed, possessiveness, conceit, jealously are not actually our enemies but are essential for our very existence.

If that is the case, why do ancient religions consider them as our enemies?

The reason lies in how we relate to them. Do we act compelled by them or do we use them as our tools?

For example, anger is generally considered to be bad. But look at how a mother acts when her beloved kid does something that can be harmful to it. She shouts, exhibits fury, and even reprimands the baby. In doing all these, she appears to be very angry with the child. But is she really? No, she often fakes those emotions just to convey the right message to the child. She is using anger to do good to the child.

Same applies to all other emotions. As long as we are not impelled by them, and we remain the real masters, they are not at all our enemies. In fact, we can use them usefully to achieve things which are not otherwise possible.

This is the first phase of mental evolution – ability to use the instincts for the betterment of not only ourselves but for others as well.

But our evolution has to go further. Let see that in the next post.

ii. Mere existence is not enough

What is the use of merely existing? We need to evolve further. Evolution enables us to better deal with uncertainties in life. Without evolution, we are at the mercy of nature and its laws that may not always be in our favor.

The trio – observation, learning and adaptation - makes us better suited for existence. They may not be essential for our existence, but definitely needed to go further. This ability comes from intelligence. And we need to be more intelligent to move on.

That is our second phase of evolution. Science is the tool in this phase of our evolution. It is not necessary that we all need to be scientists. But definitely we need to develop a scientific outlook. Otherwise, we will merely exist – and that is not too good.

But our evolution has to go further. Let see that in the next post.

iii. Science without responsibility can be bad

At one stage of evolution, humans unraveled the mysteries hidden beneath the gross nature. They literally "discovered" the vast potential of the immense energy that is hidden in the nature, in its subtle form namely the atom. We discovered atomic energy. But what happened then? Instead of using it for the benefit of humanity, we created atom bombs and busied ourselves in mass destruction and avoidable pain and suffering.

The problem is not with science. It is just that we did not use it responsibly. What we need is to temper science with morality, with ethics, with compassion. In other words, being responsible, ethical, and compassionate not only to ourselves and our people, but to all beings is the next stage of evolution. That would not only ensure our individual existence but our collective existence as well, while making the life of all more livable.

But our evolution has to go further. Let see that in the next post.

iv. Universal identity is the ultimate

In the phase zero of our existence, we remain governed by our instincts. That is how most animals and other lower level beings exist. In the next level, we evolve to use these instincts to our advantage and that of our companions. But that only ensured our existence but cannot take us further.

To move further, we need to evolve intellectually. And that is where our scientific evolution stands. But mere scientific progress is not sufficient. We need to evolve further by tempering science with morality, ethicality and compassion; that is aimed not just around us and our companions, but towards the entire universe. We need to move from 'I' to 'We'.

But that is not all. The ultimate stage of evolution is to convert this 'We' into once again 'I', the 'I' this time is broadened in its scope encompassing the entire universe. It is the universal identity. We need to identify ourselves with the entire universe.

As ancient Indian Upanishads ask "when the 'I' expands to cover the entire universe, how can anyone harm anyone else, how can anyone be afraid of anyone else? It is then; there is no 'anyone else' but just 'ME'". That is the highest level of evolution.

But this evolution probably does not happen in one step. If you want to move from New York to New Delhi, you probably need to drive to the airport, take an international flight, probably make a couple of stopovers and finally reach New Delhi. Each mode of communication is important, but none of them are ultimate. You only use them to move further. It is only the destination that is the ultimate.

32. Why do Hindus worship idols?

In the religious world, idol worship has been a contentious issue. History is replete with incidents where either a group of people holding a particular view on idol worship destroyed the sacred icons of other groups who held a different view, or looked down on them as pagans or primitive people. Recent destruction of Bamian Buddha images in Afghanistan by extremists is only a sad example.

On the other hand, modern Hindus consider idol worship as an inalienable part of their faith, so much so, that today we can't think about Hinduism without idol worship.

The intention of this series of posts is neither to justify Hindu worship of idols, nor to condemn it. My intention is to bring some interesting facts to light that would force either group to rethink on their respective stand.

In the next post, I will start with some quotes from ancient Hindu scriptures about idol worship.

i. Myth about polytheism

(Continued from "Why do Hindus worship idols?")

Before I start on idol worship, probably it is apt to clear some misconceptions about polytheism and monotheism. It is generally held that Hinduism is polytheistic and other major religions such as Judaism, Christianity, and Islam are monotheistic.

This is a misconception at least at the conceptual level. It is true that Judaism, Christianity and Islam emphasize on single God who is the supreme. Many people will be surprised that even Hinduism talks about single God. For example, one of the most ancient of Hindu scriptures namely the Veda has this to say

"They refer to as Indra, Varuna, and so on. But the fact is that the same one is called by different names by the clergy".(Rig-Veda Book I, Section 164, Verse 46)

If you look at the Upanishads (parts of Veda), the God or 'Brahma' as he/she/it is referred to, is always talked about as a single unique entity. Unlike the other world religions, this entity is considered to be not only formless, but also beyond explicit description. That is why I have used 'he/she/it' to refer to this entity as is the normal practice in these Upanishads. In one of the well known Upanishads namely the Taitarïya Upanishad, God or Brahma is defined as follows

> *"(Brahma is) that from which all the beings came into existence, that which sustains them and that into which they finally converge". (Taitarïya Upanishad, Section Bhriguvalli, Verse 1)*

And surprisingly, almost similar definition of God can be found in Quran as well as Bible!

The assertion of formlessness of God can be found throughout the ancient Hindu scriptures. I will talk more about that in the next post.

ii. You cannot know it!

(continued from "Why do Hindus worship idols?")

There is no more clear denial of the perceptible form of God than the following verses from one of the well known Hindu scriptures namely the Këna Upanishad

"That which cannot be described by words, but that from which words get revealed, know that alone as the God. And not that worshipped by people (as an object).

That which cannot be comprehended by the mind, but that by which the mind works, know that alone as the God. And not that worshipped by people (as an object).

iii. Limitations of the human mind

(Continued from "Why do Hindus worship idols?")

In the previous posts we saw how Hinduism considered the God to be not only formless but also imperceptible. The interesting question is "why do most Hindus worship idols which restrict the God to a specific form?" The answer lies partly in the well known Hindu scripture namely the Bhagavad Geetha. There it is said

"For people who are conscious of their bodies (i.e. dominated by their body), it is difficult to meditate on a formless God" (Bhagavad Geetha 12.5)

The same sentiment is expressed in the following mantra that is uttered while installing an idol in a typical Hindu temple

"I welcome you, Oh God of all Gods, who is the creator of the worlds, who is the father of all beings, who pervades the entire universe.

As an ordinary mortal with limited wisdom, I have created this form for my convenience in worshiping you. Please have mercy and make your presence felt in this image."

(Idol installation mantra in Kashyapa Silpa Sästra)

There is a difference between worshipping an idol as God, and using the idol as a medium to perceive God. This point has to be noted by both Hindus as well as others who shun idol worship.

33. Do we need to redefine science?

Recently (March 2015), the Australian National Health and Medical Research Council (NHMRC) released a statement concluding that "there is no good quality evidence to support the claim that

Homeopathy is effective in treating health conditions"

Though many Homeopathy fans are furious about this statement, the finding is by no means surprising. With its two fundamental principles – (1) whatever causes the disease can itself cure it as well, when administered in small quantities, and (2) more dilute the medicine is, the more effective it is - Homeopathy can easily be brushed aside as unscientific and illogical.

But there are several anecdotal reports claiming miraculous cures by Homeopathy. Even highly qualified allopathic doctors sometimes vouch for the efficacy of Homeopathy. In one of the cases I know, a gynecologist friend of mine who was almost bed ridden due to slip disk problem that needed immediate surgery, claims that she recovered completely by Homeopathy with no surgery. And today she is completely alright and attends to her busy medical practice.

In spite of all illogical principles and lack of concrete evidence, is there something in Homeopathy that science is yet to discover? I keep wondering. Though Homeopathy practitioners are very defensive about their system and attack with emotionally charged words anyone who questions, they seem to offer very little concrete evidence or convincing explanation about the working of their system.

I wish that they do it sooner than later. We need to either forget about Homeopathy and move ahead, or evolve our scientific approach based on new findings. I only hope one of these happens in the near future.

Continued

i. Do we need to redefine science? (continued 2)

Recently I watched a prerecorded video of a well known Yoga teacher of yester-years about how Yoga works. This supposedly Cambridge educated, one time NASA scientist was giving mysterious explanation about how Yoga works. The theory was not something new – the same "opening up of the mystical *Sushumna Naadi* by regular Yoga practice so that the dormant *Kundalini* force gets channeled through it and reaches the *Sahasrara* – all located in the *Pranic body* and 'somehow' connected to the physical body" and so on.

Many people including several well known Yoga proponents put forth this theory. What is amazing is the fact that

1. There is no verifiable evidence that such a body/naadi/force exists and such a process actually takes place.

2. Original Yoga system of Patanjali talks about none of these.
3. The theory is neither consistently nor logically defined, let alone its correctness.

In spite of these limitations, how is it that teachers after teachers talk about such mysterious things that can neither be scientifically verified, nor logically concluded, nor supported by ancient texts?

I only hope that the proponents of these theories do some serious scientific research and provide an acceptable explanation. Or suggest ways of extending our current scientific approach.

Continued

ii. Do we need to redefine science? (continued 3)

One of my readers suggested to me that I should write something on mantras that can be very useful in many ways. There are several authors who have done it before. I myself have written one book ("*A mantra to enhance your mental capabilities*"). But my effort has been to rationalize the practice and explain it in scientific terms.

But what I see now-a-days is that people seem to be least bothered about scientific basis or otherwise of several mysterious practices – be it (mono syllabic) mantra chanting or some weird hand gestures (called mudras) – that are supposed to be a cure-all for all our problems. Going by their popularity, I wonder whether science has become obsolete!

Mantra (mono syllabic) and mudra are remnants of age old tantric practices – the other three that are left out being liquor, meat and ritual sex (mantra, mudra, madira, maamsa, maithuna – the five 'M's of tantric practice). If one looks at the tantric books, the first principles of tantra are completely anti scientific – secrecy, subjectivity, total surrender to the teacher, acceptance without questioning, total rejection of reasoning, and so on.

If tantra can really achieve things as claimed, in spite of its being anti-science, it is high time that we redefine science.

Continued

iii. Do we need to redefine science? (continued 4)

The Greek philosopher Aristotle (~300 B.C.) is generally considered to be the father of modern scientific approach. Aristotle recommended observation, classification, and deduction of implications, as the sole basis of understanding nature. Or in other words, he laid emphasis on sense perception, objectivity, deduction, as we have today in our scientific approach.

Even ancient Indians considered the same – sense perception (pratyaksa), deduction (anumäna) and valid testimony (äpta väkya) - as the basis of understanding anything. But they added a rejoinder that "this approach is restricted only to knowledge related to material things. When it comes to things that are not material in nature, this approach does not work and one needs to resort to knowledge attained in super conscious state or samädhi". The statements of a person who has attained the said knowledge in such a state can be taken as "valid testimony" though it is not based on sense perception.

This is often taken as an escape route to justify all mysterious theories and explanations. In such cases we need to satisfy ourselves the credentials of the persons propagating such theories and whether they are indeed capable of transgressing the material limits. We need to be very careful before accepting such claims since in most cases they are no "valid testimony" in the strictest sense.

If it indeed turns out that such theories are true, then we need to expand the scope of science to include such findings. Definitely not otherwise.

iv. Do we need to redefine science? (continued 5)

Every person who knowingly or unknowingly propagates a mysterious theory or practice as valid may not have arrived at those theories by being at "super-conscious states" or acquired it by scientific means or from a reliable source. That being the case, it is in our interest that we ask them the following questions.

- What is the basis of their theory?
- Can they explain it logically?
- Even if they cannot explain how it works, can they at least show that it works in a sufficiently large scale, without being a chance happening? Mere anecdotal evidence – "you try it out and see it for yourself" - is not sufficient.

If answers to these questions are in the negative, then it is most likely that the theory/practice propounded is not worth considering. For all you know they can be harmful as well. Not just because of the theory, but because of the mal-intentions of the propagator of such a theory/practice.

Continued

v. Do we need to redefine science? (continued 6)

Openness is one of the cornerstones of scientific approach. The old Newtonian laws that had been taken as correct for long were revised, with no hesitation, in the light of new findings by Einstein et.al. There are many cases in the history of science where we have openly discarded old theories and accepted new ones that survived the test of scientific validity.

But in the case of several mysterious practices, this openness is a taboo. The propagators of such practices claim them to be eternally true and unquestionable. Though none of them stand the test of science, can we at least glean whatever is worth from these theories and practices by relaxing some of the stringent yardsticks of science? How do we do that?

I have suggested one way in my book "*Important missing dimensions in our current understanding of the Mind*". In that book I have considered a range of ancient philosophies that deal with Mind and reality, to see what we can learn from them. The criteria I have laid down for this purpose are the following.

We need to check whether

- The theory is self consistent: i.e. it has no internal conflicts. If the theory or practice is proposed in a book, then no part of the book should contradict any other part of the same book. Sometimes, there may be several books dealing with similar ideas and related to each other. In that case also they have to be consistent across.

If someone talks about a theory claiming it to be based on some book or sage, and if the said book or the words of the sage don't support that view or contradict that view, then also there is an internal conflict.

- The theory is unambiguous: i.e. it has clearly defined concepts. Most of the times, mysterious theories are defined in ambiguous terms. They could also be vague statements immersed in several obviously true statements that have no relation to the statement being made. Such suggestive implications often pass off as logically arrived conclusions.

- The theory is conflict free: i.e. it does not seriously conflict with well known scientific results. There are many scientific facts that have remained unchallenged for long. If some mysterious theory challenges such facts, then it better have very strong evidence. Or else it is likely to be false or fraudulent.

- The theory is useful: i.e. it provides additional insights beyond what science can, as of today, and may provide answers to some of the unanswered questions as well. Usefulness does not make the theory right. But it could be accepted as 'to be verified' theory/practice as long as it is not harmful. Many of our faiths and beliefs fall in this category. They are not proven valid, but may be useful and not known to be harmful.

Now, subject each of the things I discussed in my earlier posts – Homeopathy, Kundalini explanation to Yoga, Mantra, Mudra – to the above criteria and see how many of these survive the test?

34. Role models

When I was small, I studied in a school run by a church. Every morning we were made to assemble in the prayer hall. Before the prayers started, one of the teachers narrated a story from Bible. Though the primary purpose was religious, I am sure there was a hidden infusion of moral values in these stories. Since the stories repeated every year, we did not pay much attention to them after sometime.

Just a generation ago, I guess such practice did exist in every other community. A Hindu is probably told stories from one of their great epics, a Buddhist from Jataka stories and so on. But today these seem to have vanished and are replaced by cartoon shows and comics which are predominantly entertainment oriented.

I always wondered whether this new trend has created some void! Were those stories with underlying moral values, those idealistic role models, essential for shaping the young minds and making them better human beings?

35. The most dangerous creature on the planet!

While strolling in my friend's farm, I have often noticed that the red ants that flock the dry leaves, and inflict a rather painful sting, stop stinging once they get used to you. At times I have even encountered cobras silently crawling away with their hoods lowered, inches from my feet! No animal attacks unless it is threatened or is hungry.

I often joke that the only animal that attacks without any provocation is the human being ;-) And when I read the news on massacres and bloodshed that go on all over the world these days, in the name of religion and faith, I feel like crying on my own joke. Have we really evolved?

36. Unlimited vision

One of my readers recently asked me whether one can perceive "everything" in the world in a state of samādhi (meditation). He felt that such a thing is impossible since there are simply infinitely many things and events that keep happening at any given instant of time, not to mention those that have happened in the past.

A very interesting question indeed! Probably, this reader is prompted by such claims made by some books and authors (e.g. In "The Autobiography of a Yogi", the author Paramahamsa Yogananda talks of such experiences).

Long long ago (almost 2000 years ago), there have been serious debates in ancient India on this issue between those who claim such a possibility and those who deny such a possibility. Buddhists claim that Buddha was omniscient who could perceive everything. But the Mimamsakas (a strong group of Vedic philosophers and staunch opponents of Buddhists) tried to show in a highly *dialectical* way that no one can ever reach such a state. Their arguments were quite interesting. Some of these included

1. A person with limited perceptible capabilities can never perceive unlimited number of things.
2. Even if it is claimed that the information is perceived in a "supersensory state" like samädhi, there is no way such a person could have said that in such a state since in that state a person cannot express himself.
3. And once he comes out of samädhi, whatever he says is colored by his subjective opinions and limitations.
4. A person claiming himself to be omniscient cannot be relied upon since his

knowledge that he is omniscient has a cyclical dependency.

Having said all this, I have my reasons to believe that a person on the "threshold" of samādhi can get a glimpse of "everything" if he wishes. But most often than not, such a person is least interested in knowing any such thing. Regarding the impossibility of perceiving "everything" merely because there are infinite things – it is quite elementary knowledge that we can view a TV program from a particular channel even though there are thousands of Radio waves lingering around in the air from thousands of other channels. We merely have to tune our TV to the channel we want and the presence of other waves doesn't really matter. But the important question is – "will the desire to tune in really remain in such a state?" Most probably not.

37. Psychic powers

A few decades ago, the US government spent Billions of dollars into the research pertaining to Psychic powers. The research was carried out in top US universities by eminent scientists. At the end of the research, the scientists involved in it declared that existence of Psychic powers was beyond any doubt.

At the same time, one well known scientist, who was not part of the research process, but was a member of the two member evaluation committee questioned the way the research was carried out and concluded that the procedure was prone to erroneous conclusions and psychic powers cannot be concluded by the conducted research.

The interest in psychic powers has been there in human minds for centuries. But probably what whipped up the interest most, in recent times, are the two books – both by Indian Yoga Gurus – "Living with Himalayan Masters" by Swami Rama, and "Autobiography of a Yogi" by Paramahamsa Yogananda.

The commentator of Patanjali Yoga Sutra explained it as the power of a realized soul (Purusha) that has mastery over the matter (Prakrti). Modern Yoga teachers say that it is because of the awakening of Kundalini; while the early Buddhists said that the power was due to a "concentrated mind". Each has their own explanation, but all accept its existence.

Human mind has lot of high expectations about extraordinary phenomena, and it uses whatever is read or heard to validate its own expectations. So, even if there is glaring evidence that some Guru is just fooling the people, the mind refuses to contradict its own judgments and clings to it.

That probably explains why several pseudo Gurus thrive with their, often illogical, portrayal of psychic powers and purported methods to achieve them.

38. How far can we stretch placebo effect?

Recent research has confirmed the marvelous capabilities of placebo effect (effects caused by strong belief or expectation) on our physical as well as mental well being. I have discussed some of these in my book "How does the Mind work?"

In "How and why of Yoga and Meditation – Yoga scientifically explained" I have hinted that placebo effect could be one of the contributors to the marvelous benefits reported by the practice of Yoga postures. Though, I fully agree that benefits of Yoga postures are not all due to placebo effect.

Recently, we keep coming across several 'best sellers' that project either chanting of some monosyllable mantras or some weird hand gestures as a 'cure all' for all our problems and needs – from depression to sex! If one looks at a bit broadly, there are 'medical systems' with concepts that neither stand to logic nor have passed any large scale validation, but still have large adherents who vouch for their effectiveness.

Are we then to take placebo effect as a useful phenomenon in the long run? If we look back, human development seems to be largely due to logical reasoning rather than purely based on faith. Though we cannot altogether get us rid of faith and associated placebo effect, the question is "how far should we stretch it?"

39. Does God exist?

I have a friend – a medical doctor – who firmly believes that God does not exist. Though she does not say it openly, she puts up a front that she is agnostic. She disagrees with me when I say that acceptability of any belief rests on its utility and not necessarily on its factual correctness. I have in one of my books ("How and why of Yoga and Meditation – Yoga Scientifically explained") dealt in detail how devotional singing can be utilized to relieve one of mental stress. I have made it clear in that context that it works irrespective of the existence of God or otherwise. Just the belief is enough to make it work. I have also discussed some research findings in another of my book ("How does the mind work?") where mere beliefs seem to bestow miraculous results. In either case, the factual correctness of the belief is immaterial.

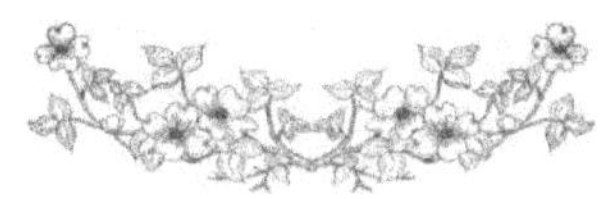

Thank you for reading my book. I hope you enjoyed reading it. Please give me your feedback through book reviews. I appreciate that very much. You may contact me through my blog at http://doctor-king-online.blogspot.com I will be happy to hear from you. If you have any specific questions or suggestions, indicate them through my blog and I will surely respond to them.

You may also be interested in reading my other books available through several online vendors.

My recent books

Following is the list of my recent books. These are available both as e-books as well as paperbacks. Some of these books are now available from one or more of online bookstores such as

Amazon, Scribd, Smashwords, Apple iBooks Store, Barnes & Noble, Sony, Kobo, Flipkart Diesel eBook Store, eBooks Eros, Baker & Taylor, Page Foundry ,WH Smith in the UK, FNAC in France and Portugul, Livraria Cultura in Brazil, Angus & Robertson in Australia, Bookworld in Australia, Indigo in Canada, Collins in Australia, Feltrinelli in Italy, Libris in the Netherlands, Paper Plus in New Zealand, Play in Great Britain, Rakuten in Japan,

Rakuten in the US, Whitcoulls in New Zealand.

Please look for them in your favorite book store. You can always use the book title in your search to see if the book is available in your favorite bookstore. I have given the appropriate links for your convenience in my blog <u>http://doctor-king-online.blogspot.com</u>

1. Hata Yoga – Myths Shattered (ASIN: B073YQL9QR)

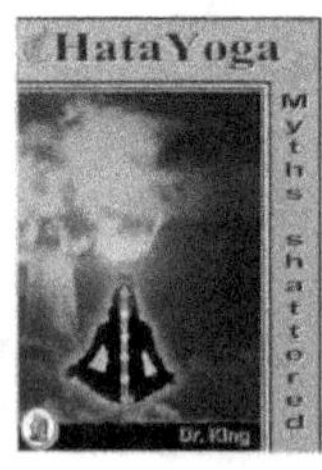

<u>Book Synopsis</u>: Hatayoga or Yoga as it is commonly referred to, is getting extremely popular. What is little known though are some of its shaky concepts that form its basis. This book makes a close scrutiny of some of these unsound concepts and comes up with amazing findings. A must read for all those who are currently practicing or intend to practice Yoga.

2. Think and be enlightened (ASIN: B071LR5WN4)

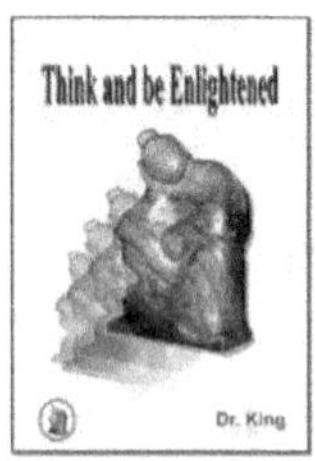

<u>Book synopsis</u>: This is a collection of thoughts in the area of Yoga, Indian philosophy, and other motivational, which make you, pander over and enrich you.

3. Mysterious Experiences: A peek beyond the confines of the Mind (ASIN: B01GLJ2F92)

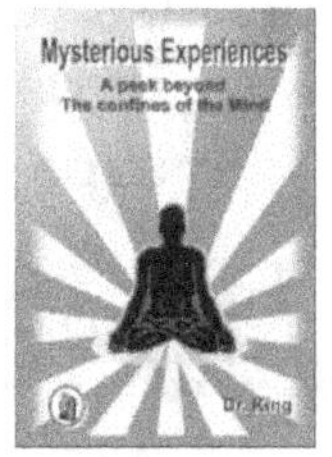

Book synopsis: This book discusses some of the interesting mysterious experiences encountered by Yoga or meditation enthusiasts It tries to provide reasoning based analysis of the situations, backed by ancient texts, and words of well known Yogis.

4. Figure Carving – The Ethnic Style: *Amazing world of possibilities* (ASIN: B017VN6AO8)

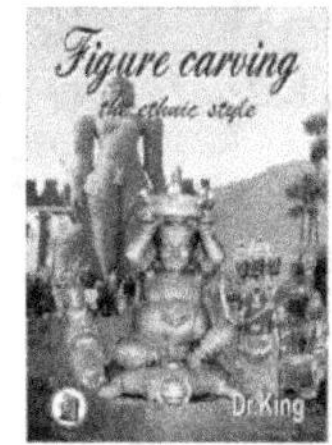

Book synopsis: This book opens up a new world of figure carving options for carving enthusiasts. It provides an unlimited number of options not only in style but also in technique backed by detailed illustrations and lots and lots of carving pictures. Add an altogether new dimension to your carving repertoire.

5. Five simple Grafting techniques best suited for most exotic fruit plants (ASIN: B00VK54IFM)

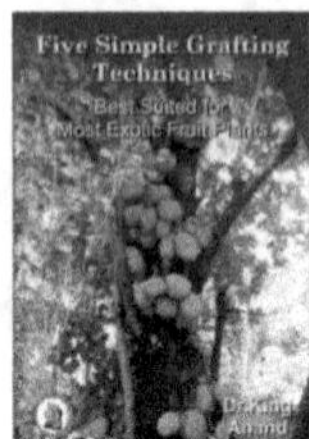

<u>Book synopsis:</u> This book describes in detail 5 most useful grafting techniques that can be used to propagate many exotic fruits. The book contains detailed illustrations, examples, fruit chart as well as root stocks and techniques well suited for these fruits.

6. How does the Mind work? (ASIN: B00J4I0374)

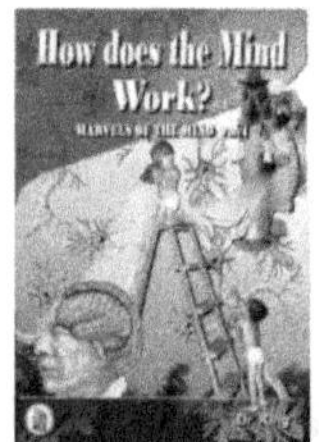

<u>Book synopsis:</u> This book explains the highly specialized subject of working of the mind in an easy to follow style using day-to-day examples. It gives latest information based on current research, focusing on key contributions.

7. Important missing dimensions in our current understanding of the Mind (ASIN: B00J4I95T6)

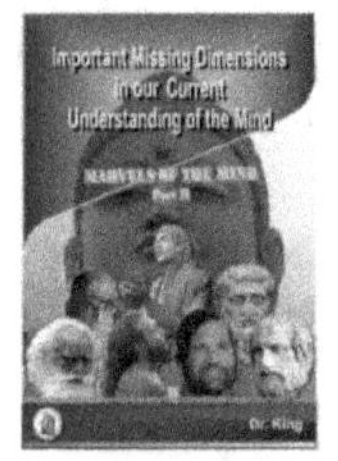

<u>Book synopsis:</u> Our current scientific achievements in understanding the working of the mind are commendable. However, in it's over insistence on objectivity science seems to have overlooked some important dimensions of the mind. There are many questions science fails to provide satisfactory answer.

Interestingly, many of these questions were addressed by ancient philosophies and probably in the true scientific spirit we should look at these philosophies with an open mind.

This book focuses on these missed dimensions and how ancient philosophies address them. A range of ancient philosophies, amazingly well conceptualized, that look at different aspects of the mind are discussed in the current book.

There is the ancient philosophy of Plato who points out the limitations of our sense perception, the elaborate psychology of ancient Buddhists that almost parallels with our scientific understanding, the philosophy of Šankara who even questions the reality of existence and the concept of domains beyond mind that are the focus of ancient Upanishads. All these, and more, are explained clearly in this second part of the series.

These philosophies compel us to rethink on our current definition of science and its approach. The book also provides a smooth transition point from science to philosophy and finally to domains beyond both these.

8. How and Why of Yoga and Meditation: *Yoga scientifically explained* (ASIN: B00TFSPTBI)

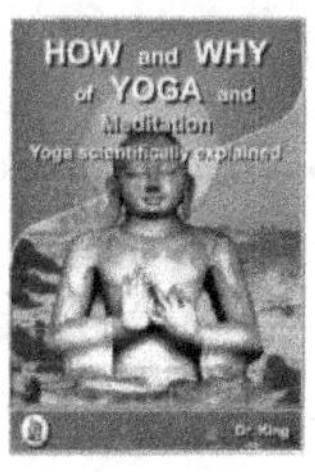

Book synopsis: This book gives a clear insight into various aspects of Yoga, while providing scientifically backed explanation about how various Yoga processes achieve their intended purposes and why they are designed that way. Such clarity is essential to understand Yoga in a more scientific manner and to realize its full potential.

The book also explains in a step by step manner how various processes of Yoga, namely the body postures, breathing techniques and meditation are performed and why each of these processes is needed to attain complete benefit of Yoga.

This book is a good guide for anyone who wants to practice Yoga.

9. Yöga Facts: Answers to some important questions about Yöga (ASIN: B00DL17A76)

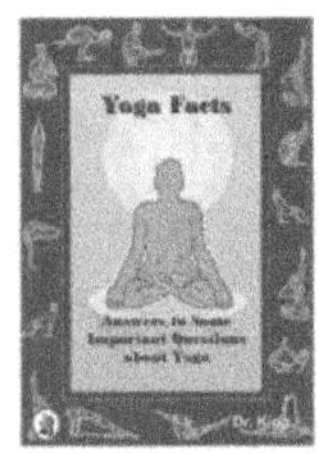

Book synopsis: Going by the large number of books on Yoga that are published and sold both through printed as well as electronic media, this ancient science seems to be very popular. While various things are propagated in the name of Yoga, there is often mismatch between expectations and achievements.

This short set of questions and answers clears some of the misconceptions about Yoga by drawing attention to the original works on Yoga dating back more than 2000 years. Questions that often arise as a result of commercially motivated propaganda are answered in a matter of fact manner. At the same time, this book reassures a sincere Yoga practitioner, that the goal is not only achievable but worth the effort.

Some of the questions discussed include - controversies due to adverse scientific findings about Yoga, why many people fail to achieve any progress in spite of sincere efforts, and so on

10. Psychology behind Yoga: Lesser known insights into the ancient science of Yoga (ASIN: B00BFRDOPA)

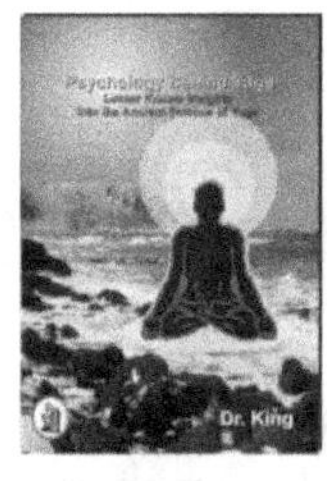

Book synopsis: Though Yöga is well known as a process to achieve the ultimate realization, not much attention is paid to its psychological underpinnings. This book builds up the theory behind Yoga based on descriptions given in ancient texts such as Yoga sutra of Patanjali (~200 B.C.) and Sänkhya Kärika of Isvara Krshna (~300 A.D.). This understanding is essential to get a complete grasp of the Yöga process.

This book clearly explains the concept of mind as defined in Yoga Sutra and Sänkhya Kärika, various states this mind can be in, and how by a step by step process the mind can be nudged into the ultimate desirable state namely the Samadhi. It discusses various hindrances one encounters while going through this process as well as how these can be overcome. As often mistaken, samädhi is not a single state but a series of progressive states one goes through as one progresses into the Yoga practice. This book explains those stages both with reference to the original sources as well as through simple analogies.

The ultimate state of Yoga, namely the niruddha state of mind is also very well explained, its implications and what exactly happens in that stage.

11. Ancient Wisdom – Modern Viewpoints: Interesting picks from ancient Indian scriptures (ASIN: B00BBDASC0)

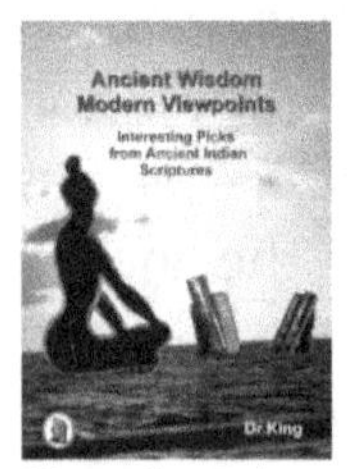

Book synopsis: This book captures the essence of ancient Indian scriptures, analyzing them from today's point of view. The scriptures selected are mainly the eleven Upanishads (parts of Vedic literature), Bhagavad Geetha (most important book of Indian philosophy) and the Manu Smrthi (one of the most ancient law books by Manu). All these scriptures were composed more than 2500 years ago and influence the Indian way of life even to this day. In addition to these primary scriptures, this book also cross references several other ancient Indian scriptures such as Yoga Sutra of Patanjali, Sänkhya Kärika, Närada Bhakti sutra, and Dammapada.

Some of the key aspects of each of these three main scriptures – Upanishads, Bhagavad Geetha and Manu Smrthi - are picked and presented in 6 short, crisp articles. While writing these articles, the original Sanskrit texts are relied upon with minimal re-interpretation.

Adequate references to the original Sanskrit verses are given in most places, to impart authenticity to the rendering. To help the readers who may not be familiar with Sanskrit, simple English translations of these verses are also provided.

This is an ideal book for anyone who wants to have a quick overview of most of the ancient Indian scriptures. The book gives a wealth of information and surely a key to the treasure of ancient Indian scriptures.

12. A Mantra to enhance your mental capabilities (ASIN: B00EV496UG)

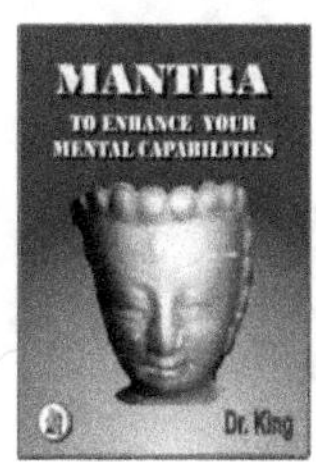

Book synopsis: For thousands of years, millions of people have taken advantage of one mantra which is believed to enhance the mental capabilities. Though it is used even today, it has become a prerogative of a small minority of people and seems to be going into the oblivion. The ravages of time has seriously rendered this potent mantra into an article of religious faith and deep rooted superstition, depriving the vast majority from realizing its benefits.

This book opens up this mantra to all those who are desirous of enhancing their mental capabilities. It discusses various aspects of this mantra and explains in a step by step fashion how anyone can take advantage of this mantra

13. Around the Mind

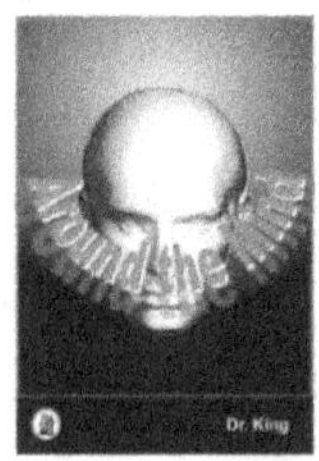

<u>Book synopsis:</u> Mind may probably be the most intriguing thing that has fascinated human beings, philosophers as well as the scientists, for thousands of years. This book summarizes our current scientific views on the Mind, the questions that arise due to that view, the efforts by ancient philosophies to address these questions and probably a possibility of going beyond the realms of current scientific approach.

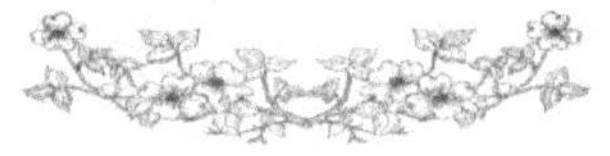